The Snowshoe Experience

The Snowshoe Experience

Gear up & discover
the wonders of winter
on snowhoes

Claire Walter

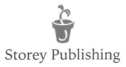

Storey Publishing

The mission of Storey Publishing is to serve our customers by publishing practical information that encourages personal independence in harmony with the environment.

Edited by Michael Robbins and Sarah Guare
Cover and text design by Wendy Palitz
Front cover photographs © Jim Gipe
Back cover photographs © David Stoecklein/CORBIS (top inset),
    Jack Sullivan/Alamy Images (bottom inset)
Illustrations © Elayne Sears
Text production by Jennifer Jepson Smith
Indexed by Eileen Clawson

Printed in the United States by Versa Press
10 9 8 7 6 5 4 3 2 1

Library of Congress Cataloging-in-Publication Data
Walter, Claire.
  The snowshoe experience : gear up & discover the wonders of winter on snowshoes / Claire Walter.
      p. cm.
  Includes index.
  ISBN 1-58017-541-4 (pbk. : alk. paper)
  1. Snowshoes and snowshoeing. I. Title.
GV853.W34 2004
796.92—dc22
                                    2004016567

Contents

Foreword

Winter is my favorite time of year. The air becomes crisp and cool. The sky turns from a deep blue to a soft white, and the snow flies. Slowly, the ground is covered and all you can see is a never-ending fluffy, soft white playground. Being the active, adventurous person I am, the first thing I do when the snow flies is to strap on my snowshoes and head out to explore. Snowshoeing provides the opportunity to enjoy the peace and serenity of the outdoors in winter, while at the same time taking you to new levels of fitness.

Originally, snowshoes were an essential winter tool, used to get from one place to another and to gather and hunt food during snowy conditions. Snowshoeing has since turned into a recreational activity and sport for all ages and abilities. I have seen children as young as two or three out snowshoeing with their great-grandparents, who were over 90. Snowshoeing is also a competitive sport, with over 400 events and thousands of participants every year in North America alone. Snowshoeing provides competitive opportunities for winter sports enthusiasts internationally.

I am not only a competitive athlete, but also a personal trainer who has worked with all sorts of people who want to become healthier and stronger. Just about anyone can snowshoe — and benefit from it. That's a message that I try to pass on to my clients and to anyone else who is interested in this wonderful winter activity. Whatever your level of interest and fitness, *The Snowshoe Experience* will provide you with much knowledge, sound advice, and many pointers so that you can better enjoy your experience.

I first met Claire at a snowshoe clinic that I was presenting in Boulder, Colorado. She had extensive knowledge of some of the best places to go snowshoeing in the state. I was impressed! I knew instantly that she shared the same passion for snowshoeing as I did. She enjoys snowshoeing more for the exploration and beauty, while I focus more on the fitness and competitive side of the sport. Claire shares her extensive knowledge in this guide. So remember her pointers, and when the snow flies, get out there and enjoy!

— Danelle Ballangee
2002 National Snowshoe Champion; 2002 Adventure Racer of the Year; competitor in the Ironman Triathlon; and winner of more than 100 snowshoe races

Introduction

Snowshoeing can mean the difference between loving and loathing winter. It is a passport to the joys of the winter outdoors that is within comfortable reach of anyone. It is winter's answer to walking and hiking, which have been pegged as America's most popular outdoor leisure activities. It crosses boundaries of age, fitness level, outdoor experience, and personal ambition. Snowshoeing is just about the easiest and most versatile of all sports. The basic technique is so simple that it really doesn't require much instruction. It essentially involves strapping on snowshoes, putting one foot in front of the other, and walking. In fact, most instructions are less about how to do it than how to adjust the gear.

With snowshoes, you can explore virtually any place where there is snow. These big feet attach to your own smaller ones for hassle-free access to the white winter world. The limitations are those you put on yourself, such as how fit you are, what your comfort level is in the outdoors, and how you feel about guided touring versus the quiet companionship of just a good friend or two. Snowshoeing is a tranquil activity, yet it can be a sociable one. The learning curve is minimal, the rewards come practically with the first step, and the risk of injury is one of the lowest of all outdoor sports. This is a multi-generational activity, one which parents can do with their children and adults can do with their parents. Snowshoeing in the backcountry with a group of companions is not just a winter pleasure, but a safety measure as well.

One of the major benefits of this sport is that snowshoers are literally *out there*. They are not driving around a parking lot searching for the closest entrance to the mall. They are not curled up in a lounge chair, exercising their remote-control-operating fingers. They are out moving in the fresh air, and they are healthier for it. When Bruce Carey, a 40-year-old Vail, Colorado, attorney who thought of himself as reasonably trim, went for a medical checkup, he got the scare of his life. "My internist said, 'Exercise or insulin,'" he recalls. "I took up snowshoeing. I lost 3 inches from my middle — and I didn't need insulin." Carey became a snowshoe-racing enthusiast and took a part-time job leading snowshoe tours at the Beaver Creek Cross-Country and Snowshoe Center. He is one of the growing number of evangelists for the many health benefits of outdoor exercise, in winter as well as in summer.

A lot of Americans would do well to heed Carey's message. With our unfortunate predilection for processed foods and fast foods that are high in calories, sugar, and fats, we are, tragically, becoming a nation of plus-sized citizens with all the attendant health risks. The chances of contracting diabetes, cancer, heart disease, and cardiovascular disease are reduced when weight is reduced, and it's no secret that exercise is a key component in weight control. Snowshoeing is an ideal winter activity for people who are overweight, out of shape, or simply uncoordinated.

In fact, snowshoes provide such a stable platform and snowshoeing is so easy that as a Winter Special Olympics event, it is manageable even by individuals with extreme physical and developmental challenges who can navigate a short, straightforward course. Whatever activity on the walking-to-running continuum that you do on bare ground in summer is possible in winter on snowshoes. If you are a casual walker who likes an occasional leg stretch in the fresh air, you can strap on snowshoes and amble across a snow-covered meadow in a city park, up an unplowed country lane, or along an urban recreation trail. If you are a sturdy hiker, strap those hiking boots into a pair of snowshoes, and hit your favorite trail. If you are an ardent backpacker, outfit yourself with subzero gear and try winter camping, the epitome of backcountry self-sufficiency and solitude. If you are a runner, you won't find a better way to stay in shape through the cold months than to run on snow-shoes, and if you like to compete, there's a full calendar of winter races in the north country.

Most of us are neither Special Olympians nor backcountry addicts nor gonzo runners, and snowshoeing fills that large lump on the bell curve that represents most people's interests and abilities. Its low-key nature is ideal for those of us who are over 50 and want an easy way to enjoy winter, bond with nature, and get some exercise. Think of the options. As a snowshoer, you can follow a well-marked trail at a cross-country ski center or Alpine ski area, amble along a hiking trail, or mean-der through a local park path where it's impossible to get lost or confused. You can roam around in the confined area of a snowed-in campground to get the feel of snowshoeing or wander down a snow-covered logging or mining road that may be closed to vehicles in winter. You can enjoy snowshoeing with your family or a group of friends, or join a guided naturalist tour to learn about the winter world. And again, whatever your starting point may be, whether couch potato or endurance runner, plugging snowshoeing into your winter life will make you fitter, healthier, stronger, and fleeter.

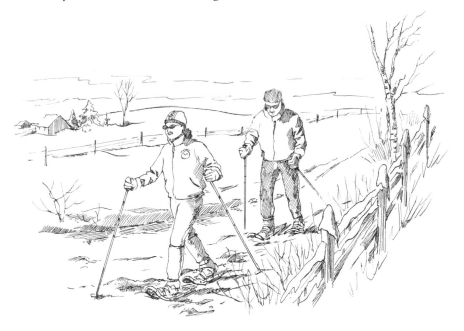

My own introduction to snowshoeing came one winter when I signed up for a ranger-guided tour through the Mariposa Grove of Giant Sequoias in Yosemite National Park. The snowshoes were classic wooden, tennis racquet-style models, which felt heavy and awkward for my height and weight. The wet snow, nicknamed Sierra Cement, wadded up between the snowshoes and my boot soles. It hardened under my feet and felt as if there were baseballs under my arches. I struggled along like the proverbial drunken sailor until I could hardly stand up. Then I stopped, removed my snowshoes, and chipped away rock-hard clumps so I could continue walking or, I should say, waddling, because that was how my awkward gait felt.

Even with the challenge of that equipment and that particular type of snow, I could feel the inherent advantages of snowshoes. After the ranger had explained the ecology of the sequoia forest, I stomped off alone, away from the group, to be awed by the place without worrying about sinking knee-deep into the snow. Looking up at those majestic trees was humbling, and so was snowshoeing itself. I felt awkward on those big, flopping snowshoes, but I gamely waddled along, knocking the snow clumps off my boots now and again. I ran out of steam just about the time that the tour, designed for neophytes like me, was over. Still, even in my discomfort, I felt intuitively snowshoes had great potential, if someone would only perfect them. The potential I felt has now been realized, with the development of modern, lightweight, easy-to-use snowshoes. What is probably the oldest ancient form of travel over snow has become an increasingly popular winter recreation. I still treasure the freedom and ease of snowshoeing that I sensed that first day. I treasure the sheer pleasure and good exercise that snowshoeing provides, as well. If you are a snowshoer, you probably remember your first time too. If you haven't yet been bitten by the snowshoe bug, surely you will feel it when you are.

one

History 101

Where snowshoeing has been & where it's going

Snowshoeing is one of the oldest snow sports and one of the newest. At the end of the 20th century and the beginning of the 21st, the low-cost, low-key sport of snowshoeing enjoyed a surge and became America's fastest-growing winter sport. But its history goes back through the millennia. Snowshoes' origins are shrouded in the misty days of prehistory and distant places. Experts have pegged 4000 B.C. or so as the time the earliest ones were fashioned as a more efficient way for people in northerly climates to move across the snow. The purpose of snowshoes at this time was not, of course, for recreation, but rather for transportation.

Some archaeologists believe that the earliest snowshoes were wood, bark, or stiffened rawhide formed into circles or ovals, while others believe that they were solid slabs of wood lashed to the foot with leather, vines, or reeds. Most agree that they probably were first made in central Asia. It is therefore not inconceivable that the people who crossed the Bering land bridge to North America did so on snowshoes. It has also been said that Alexander the Great's soldiers later moved across deep snow on wood hoops with platforms of woven rush to provide flotation.

Over the centuries, snowshoes changed. The native peoples of the arctic region — those early North Americans whose ancestors might well have come to this continent on rudimentary snowshoes — continued to use them. Their descendants moved south into the Great Plains where winter is forceful and intense, as well as into the snowy, forested zones that we call the North Woods. The trappers, traders, hunters, explorers, surveyors, woodsmen, and ranchers who subsequently trekked westward adapted these practical designs. While visiting the Museum of the Rockies in Bozeman, Montana, I was quite captivated by artist George Catlin's images of Indian hunters on snowshoes bringing down deer and even bison in the 1830s.

These north-country travelers and dwellers slowly refined the concept and developed finely crafted wood-frame models, often of ash with rawhide webbing, and eventually added crossbars for lateral stability and shape retention. They also discovered that long-tailed models were an improvement over simple oval shapes for tracking straight, and they tinkered with the part that actually holds the foot onto the snowshoe, what we today call the binding.

There was some 19th- and early 20th-century blurring of the line between snowshoes and skis, though technically, the former were usually understood to be webbed for walking, while the latter were longer, narrower, and made of solid wood for sliding. But then recreational use increased and, around the turn of the last century, snowshoeing as we know it became a popular leisure-time activity. The Canadian Snowshoer's Union was founded in 1907 to systemize the activities of some 60 snowshoeing clubs that had popped up in eastern Canada. These spiffy organizations had uniforms, band music, an almost militaristic hierarchy topped by officers in club leadership positions, and a schedule of snowshoe races. Early 1900s races took place over various distances on packed-snow oval tracks, much like horse races, foot races, and long-track speed skating events, and these races became a winter-carnival staple at communities across the snowbelt. The popularity of snowshoeing and snowshoe clubs drifted southward into New England, and in 1925, Lewiston, Maine, hosted the first International Snowshoe Convention to celebrate the joy of this hearty winter sport. Through the 1930s, community, fraternal, and local sports organizations put on snowshoe outings, which were popular in many locales. Seventy years after the Canadians founded their first snowshoeing association, the United States Snowshoe Association was established. USSSA has morphed from a largely recreational organization into the sanctioning body for the growing number of serious snowshoe races. Snowshoemag.com is a current on-line snowshoe publication aimed at elite snowshoers and enthusiasts alike. For a time, an enthusiasts' magazine called *The Snowshoer* was published. Check out the Web sites provided in the Resources section (pages 131–132).

During the late 19th and early 20th century, however, snowshoes were usually more utilitarian than recreational. One of the most amazing tales of winter survival and selfless heroism took place in 1897, when eight whaling ships were trapped in the arctic ice near Point Barrow, Alaska's nothernmost settlement. Ship owners, concerned that the 265 crew members would starve before the spring breakup, appealed to President William McKinley for a relief expedition. The task fell to the United States Coast Guard, which dispatched the cutter *Bear*, from Port Townsend, Washington, in late November. At Cape Vancouver, Alaska, which was as far as the cutter could go that late in the year, the captain assigned a shore party to mount a rescue. The plan was to enlist the aid of natives, buy a herd of reindeer, and drive the animals 1,500 miles to the stranded whalers. The men set off on December 16, 1897, using dog sleds, reindeer-pulled sleds that were nothing like the Santa Claus fantasy, snowshoes, and skis. On March 29, 1898, after fighting brutal temperatures, fierce blizzards, and the long, lonely arctic nights, the rescuers arrived at Point Barrow and brought 382 reindeer to feed the stranded men.

Though little known, this story, in which snowshoes played a crucial part, seems to me on a par with two more famous winter feats. The story of Captain Ernest Shackleton's terrifying Antarctic expedition is well known. Books have been written and films made about Shackleton's astonishing feat of saving every single crewmember aboard his ship, the *Endurance,* when it was crushed by ice in 1915. Another well-known story is the heroic 1925 dogsled relay, during which 20 mushers and their teams raced 674 miles from the Nenana railroad station to Nome, Alaska, to deliver anti-diphtheria serum to the stricken village. The feat inspired the legendary Iditarod dogsled race. Balto, the lead dog on the team that carried the serum the last 63 miles into Nome, is memorialized with a statue in New York City's Central Park.

Snowshoes are footnotes to military history as well. Military snowshoe training on the North American continent took place in the mid-18th century, when Robert Rogers, credited with establishing what are now the Army Rangers, changed the way English colonists did battle. In 1758, while other units were bivouacked in winter quarters, his Rangers used snowshoes, sleds, and even ice skates to send scouting parties and raiders against the French and Indian foes. Canada's Hudson's Bay Company, established in the 17th century to collect fur for export to Mother England, evolved over the years to become the country's most comprehensive and best-known department store chain. Within days after receiving an urgent order for special winter equipment for British soldiers who expected to see winter action in northern Europe during World War II, the Winnipeg store began shipping 7,400 pairs of snowshoes, 10,000 pairs of rubber boots, and 7,000 pairs of moccasins overseas. Tubbs, one of America's pioneer snowshoe manufacturers, made the snowshoes for the Tenth Mountain Division, the legendary United States Army unit that trained for mountain warfare at Camp Hale in the high country near Tennessee Pass in Colorado. The men of the Tenth practiced summer and winter maneuvers, learning to be climbers, mountaineers, and skiers. Less well known was the division's use of snowshoes in the deep snows of the high Rockies, particularly by the artillery and heavy-weapons platoons. The Tenth distinguished itself with a heroic and successful mountaineering assault against German forces in Italy, and veterans of the division are widely credited with launching America's post-World War II ski resort boom.

After the war, winter training continued as Battalion Level 38th Mountain/Winter Warfare Survival Group carried on where the Tenth had left off. "Our gear consisted of skis, ski boots, snowshoes, shoe packs, a three-section sleeping bag, mountain tent, mountain stove, extra outer and inner wear, ski parka, overcoat parka, white camo outfit, two sets of gloves (one with a trigger finger), rations, two canteens, cartridge belt (with ammo), mess kit, bayonet, M1 rifle and other combat weapons, along with an assortment of survival equipment," recalls one anonymous veteran on a Web site devoted to the 38th Mountaineers' legacy. "The men carried over 90 pounds of combat and survival gear as well as special winter clothes and boots. We did it all on foot with skis and snowshoes. It's on record that the men who trained at Camp Hale during 1947–1948 were trained as Special Forces." The Tenth Mountain Division's experience in World War II and the 38th Mountaineers' continuation carried over into the Korean conflict, where the United States Army units trained on the Japanese island of Hokkaido in winter survival skills, including how to use snowshoes.

The United States military still trains for winter warfare on snowshoes and other gear. The Army National Guard operates the Mountain Warfare School near Jericho, Vermont, where Army Reserve, National Guard, and others attend two-week winter mountaineering school. The United States Marines operate the Northern Warfare Training Center near Bridgeport, California, in the High Sierra range. The Marine Corps Mountain Warfare Training Center (MCMWTC) is a remote and isolated post located nearly 6,800 feet above sea level. Established in 1951 to provide cold-weather training for troops bound

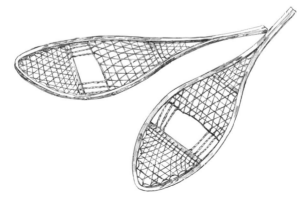

beavertail snowshoes (without bindings)

for Korea, the training center operated on a full-time basis until 1967, when it was placed in caretaker status as a result of the Vietnam War, in which winter warfare was certainly not an issue. It was reactivated to full-time command in 1976. The Army's Northern Warfare Training Center at Fort Wainwright, 30 miles from Delta Junction, Alaska, prepares troops to function successfully in brutal arctic, subarctic, and mountain environments and the harshest winter conditions. The military now uses tungsten snowshoes manufactured in camouflage white, as were the woodies used by the men of the Tenth — but I'm getting ahead of the story.

The Advent of Aluminum

With peace and, later, the arrival of lightweight metal on the snowshoeing scene, everything changed. As I had experienced at Yosemite (see Introduction, page 1), those traditional snowshoes required a modicum of skill, whether the snowshoer was using them for utilitarian or recreational purposes. Not only did I have problems with icy snowballs forming under my boots, but the technique of snowshoeing itself didn't come naturally to me. I remember that those woodies, which probably should have been retired to become decorative objects over someone's mountain-home fireplace, were large and heavy. Even if my memory of what those snowshoes looked like is inaccurate, I am sure that they felt awkward on my feet. I've since learned that long snowshoes with tails require a lengthening of the stride and wide snowshoes require a wide-gait waddle, but that was not intuitive to me.

After the slow evolution during which wooden models and also snowshoe bindings were steadily improved, the late 20th century witnessed a true revolution in snowshoe design. A handful of innovators (the winter sports equivalent of garage computer tinkerers) made dramatic technical advances, primarily in designing lightweight, easy-to-use aluminum-frame snowshoes.

The first of these innovators was a pair of technically inclined mountaineering brothers from Washington named Gene and Bill

Prater. Though primarily a farmer, Gene had studied engineering and had learned about aircraft materials while working at Boeing. They used snowshoes for winter climbing approaches. It didn't take long for them to recognize the drawbacks of the clumsy wooden models that were not suitable for demanding ascents and descents. In the early 1950s, the Praters set out to "fix" snowshoes, initially by modifying World War II Army surplus models. First, they tried to improve traction by wrapping extra rawhide around the wooden frame. Then, they installed a serrated metal bar underfoot, which really helped grip the snow surface. They found that making the tail area smaller minimized or even eliminated the wearying waddle gait, which helped them walk with a more natural stride.

But ultimately, they decided on a whole new approach to combat the large wooden snowshoes' inherent flaws: a tendency of the retaining straps to slip off the foot at times that were inopportune for mountaineering, a lack of traction while ascending or descending, and exhaustion and soreness brought on by the straddle walk. In the early 1970s, Gene's experiments produced the first snowshoes made of modern materials. He settled on a frame design smaller than the prevalent wooden models of the day, oval in shape, and constructed of an aluminum alloy. Instead of the traditional webbing, he made a deck from neoprene sheet laced onto the metal frame. The Praters formed a company and called it Sherpa Design after the Sherpa Climbing Club, whose members tackled Cascade mountains and were happy to lend the club's name to the Praters' new-fangled mountaineering snowshoes.

Sherpa Design's Mountain line debuted in 1974, and if you can ever find a pair, they are probably now more collectible than a wall full of antique woodies. The brothers' two decades of designing, testing, redesigning, retesting, and perfecting this revolutionary snowshoe resulted in built-in features that were dazzling to anyone who had struggled with conventional snowshoes. The synthetic decking provided more flotation within a smaller frame than the old snowshoes. The new type of binding easily adjusted to any size boot. Anodizing the tubular aluminum kept the wet Cascade snow from sticking to the frames. A hinged steel rod underfoot coupled with the conventional toe hole enabled the wearer to move his or her boot toe through the plane of the snowshoe without wobbling. Well after Sherpa had set the standard for snowshoes, Eric Prater continued to operate the family farm and to design snowshoes under the Prater label to carry on the family tradition.

In 1908, Walter Tubbs, of Norway, Maine, began fashioning the snowshoes that carry his name. Tubbs outfitted Admiral Richard Byrd's South Pole expeditions in the 1930s with snowshoes, sleds, and even snowshoe furniture to make camp more civilized and comfortable. Tubbs later relocated his firm to Vermont, and a new owner eventually affiliated it with the Stowe Canoe Company, a pairing of two classic outdoor gear brands.

A chap named Bill Perkins carried the banner of aluminum-frame snowshoes into the Rocky Mountain region. A triathlete living and training in the cold, high, snow-laden clime of Leadville, Colorado, he wanted to be able to run outdoors year-round and also to compete in a quirky competition in nearby Vail known as the Mountain Man Winter Triathlon. Working in the mid-1980s, Perkins meshed the Prater-type materials technology of lightweight aluminum with the traditional beavertail shape. This new model, called the Redtail, became the "flagship," if you will, of the Redfeather line that debuted in 1988. This high-performance showstopper combined high-strength aircraft-quality aluminum (anodized in a sexy red) with decking and toe cord made of Hypalon, the rugged synthetic fabric used for whitewater rafts. The first year, Perkins and his then-partner Alan Moye made 100 pairs, selling half to whoever could be persuaded to buy them and giving half to leading endurance athletes. These picky runners quickly adopted this lightweight, ergonomically friendly, high-performance snowshoe. Production tripled the next year and doubled again by 1991 to 600 pairs. Redtails had established themselves as the brand to beat on the nascent snowshoe racing circuit.

Like many innovators, Perkins was more of a creative force than a business brain. The Perkins-Moye partnership dissolved, Redfeather changed hands several times, and Perkins was ultimately bought out of the company he had founded. "The best days were when I didn't know what I was doing, and we were doomed," Perkins once told a reporter. He consulted for Tubbs in the development of their aluminum-frame snowshoes and also for other snowshoe makers, but Redfeather remains his greatest legacy to the snowshoeing sport. Meanwhile, Redfeather continued fine-tuning its pioneering easy-to-use bindings, added a narrower women-specific binding, and refined the race binding. Other companies making aluminum-frame snowshoes came along with their own innovations in shape, materials, and binding designs.

Mountain Safety Research, which started as a one-man operation in the 1960s to create safe, high-quality climbing equipment, brought more new ideas about materials and design to snowshoeing. In 1995, Seattle-based MSR introduced a one-piece snowshoe of molded plastic that incorporated the frame and the decking into a single unit. Several other snowshoe makers quickly followed and brought out variations on the theme of a one-piece plastic shoe. Meanwhile, MSR also initiated the use of an elastic material for bindings to make them easier to put on and remove, tail extenders for added flotation in deep snow, and a heel lift for greater ease and comfort while ascending steep slopes.

It may have taken centuries for wooden slabs to evolve into more functional wooden snowshoes and a couple of decades for the Praters to make the shift to truly functional aluminum-frame models, but other innovations happened quickly once Sherpa and other pioneering companies had established the new aluminum standard for snowshoe design. These revolutionary designs took hold in the '80s and '90s, just as millions of Americans had rediscovered fitness and the joy of being outdoors and, in some cases, sought an alternative winter diversion to the high-energy, high-cost sports of Alpine skiing and snowboarding. According to the National Association of Sporting Goods, 444,000 pairs of snowshoes were sold in 1994, skyrocketing to 640,000 the following year and more than a million the year after that. Between 1998 and

2003, snowshoeing reportedly grew 92 percent and the total number of American snowshoers was estimated at 5.9 million.

According to figures compiled by SnowSports Industries America, something on the order of 1 million Americans identify themselves as snowshoers, meaning that nearly 5 million more may do it occasionally. And just who are these snowshoers? They are in their years of prime activity, with 44.5 percent between the ages of 25 and 44. Nearly 10 percent are between the ages of 7 and 11. If you think of snowshoeing as a "girlie activity," think again. SIA says that nearly 60 percent of all snowshoers are men.

For decades, nearly all of the snowshoes used in North America were actually designed and manufactured in North America. That is changing now, too. K2, Inc., originally a ski and later snowboard manufacturer, moved into snowshoes in a big way. In 2003, it acquired WinterQuest, Inc., the parent company of Tubbs and Atlas, two long-running snowshoe brands that are said to command about 80 percent of the worldwide snowshoeing market, and soon began to move its manufacturing overseas.

To say that there is a "snowshoe industry" in the same breath with, say, the "steel industry," "automotive industry," or "publishing industry," is, of course, hyperbole. But it is no exaggeration that snowshoeing has matured well beyond the visionary basement innovators and garage fabricators of the past. Snowshoes today are designed in modern ways, systematically tested, and manufactured with precision to last and last. Meanwhile, Americans have responded, and despite the well-documented national migration to the sunbelt, unprecedented numbers of people who love winter have discovered snowshoeing and established their place in the backcountry as well as on established trails. I'm one of them — and hopefully, you will be too.

two

Gearing Up

Equipment for the Simple Sport of Snowshoeing

A t its most basic, snowshoeing requires only the snowshoes them-selves, sturdy footwear that keeps the feet warm and dry, and proper winter clothing. Snowshoes are made for one purpose: To allow a person to move across the snow without sinking down deeply. From the outset, they became as functional as other basic human innovations, such as the wheel, the pulley, the spear, and the vessel for carrying water. Each one was developed to make life easier for the people whose intuition and inventiveness brought them forth, but over time, these simple solutions to basic problems were refined into objects of consid-erable grace and, often, beauty. So it is with the classic wooden snow-shoe, often dismissed as being old-fashioned. In truth, it is a graceful and aesthetic link to the sport's past.

Traditional wooden snowshoes have been around a long time — cen-turies, in fact — and have passed the test of time. The common denominator was a braced bentwood frame with webbing or lacing of rawhide or other material to provide flotation over the snow, some kind of strap system to secure the snowshoe to the boot, and a pliable strip, called the toe cord, that allowed the snowshoer to walk easily. A hole under the forefoot allowed the foot to flex with every step. A turned-up tip prevented the front of the snowshoe from diving into loose snow. There's a lot of terminology related to these antiques that you

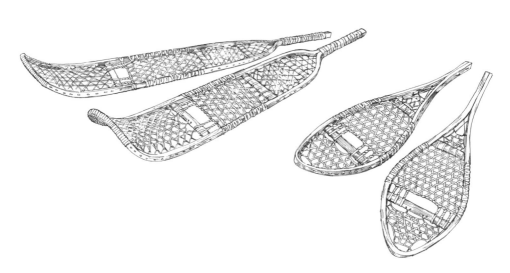

Yukon snowshoes *Algonquin snowshoes*

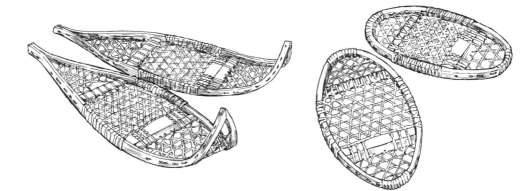

Ojibwa snowshoes *Bearpaw snowshoes*

probably won't need to know unless you find yourself gravitating toward the shapes and materials that represent snowshoeing's heritage. Snowshoes gradually evolved into four basic and distinct shapes that are associated with particular regions and particular types of snow and terrain. Some styles have two or more names. Whether you are an iconoclastic Luddite who prefers the old styles or, like most snowshoers, feel more comfortable with the new designs, the following information will at least clarify some of snowshoeing's heritage.

The **Yukon, Alaskan, Pickerel,** or **trail** style is the giant among snowshoes. This oblong shoe, usually from 4 to 5 feet long and about a foot wide, has a turned-up toe and long tail for tracking straight over flat open land and for added stability. This style was developed for use in deep, heavy snow, especially over nonmountainous, open terrain, yet it is also well suited to descending steep slopes when the snow is soft.

The **Algonquin, beavertail, Maine, Michigan,** or **Huron** snowshoe is a foot or two shorter but a couple of inches wider than the Yukon. It also has a long tail, but the toe is relatively flat. Measuring from 10 to 20 inches in width and from 30 to 40 inches in length, this type became most popular with Eastern snowshoers because it is good for hill ascents. It is also the closest design from the wooden-shoe era to the modern notion of an all-terrain snowshoe.

The **Ojibwa,** designed in central Canada where deep snow blankets wide-open tracts, is a large snowshoe. It is known for two characteristics: a pointed, turned-up toe and a long tail that is also turned up. Also, while most wooden snowshoe frames are made of a single piece of curved wood, the Ojibwa is made of two pieces that are joined together at both the heel and the toe. This snowshoe can be as small as 9 by 36 inches or as beefy as 12 by 60 inches.

Finally, the **bearpaw** snowshoe is a short, wide, and fairly flat oval suitable for even ground. Originally, bearpaws ranged from 14 by 36 inches to 12 by 30 inches; later, the most common bearpaw was a modified model sometimes called the **Green Mountain bearpaw,** which measured about 10 by 36 inches. The bearpaw is good for kicking steps in the snow during steep ascents. Some later modifications incorporated a tapered tail design to help the snowshoes track and a raised tip to clear deep snow, as well as size adjustments that made them suitable for travel through underbrush and thickets.

Native peoples of the North American snowbelt — the Algonquin, Huron, and Iroquois in the East, the Inuits and Eskimos of the arctic region, the Arapaho on the Western Plains, and other groups — were particularly adept at both making and using snowshoes. When traders, trappers, explorers, loggers, hunters, and settlers began fanning out across the north country, they adopted the native practice of traveling over the snow on snowshoes. During World War II, Allied troops readied for battle at northerly latitudes by training on snowshoes large enough to support a soldier carrying a heavy pack. Tubbs produced hundreds of thousands of pairs of big white beavertail snowshoes, and for years, Army surplus stores sold them to anyone strong and energetic enough to use them. Generations of snowshoers learned, by trial and error, what worked well and what worked less well under various snow and terrain conditions. These long-running trial-and-error experiments resulted in adaptations which have been translated into modern material and incorporated in the metal-frame snowshoes that are dominant in North America today.

Though Tubbs' aluminum-frame snowshoes were among the first in the sport's modern renaissance, the Vermont company is also tending the flame of wooden snowshoe making. Stowe's Joan Scribner-Lemieux is the one-woman fire tender. This great-grandmother is New England's last remaining snowshoe lacer. It is an honor to watch her sure hands practice this traditional craft. She first soaks cowhide to soften it and then slices it into thin strips. She clamps a bentwood frame of sturdy white ash onto a rack and begins to thread the flexible cowhide through it. With a large hook, she crosses the strip back upon itself, keeping it flat in places for flotation and twisting it in other places for strength. When she needs to splice two strips together, she cuts slits near the ends and subtly knots them together. It takes a little over an hour to lace a pair of snowshoes, after which they are dipped in varnish to seal the wood and the cowhide. Finally, modern bindings are attached.

Joan was a snowshoer long before she started making snowshoes. "For years, I worked with the Girl Scouts," she recalls, "and every year, we took a winter camping trip on snowshoes. It was great to watch the girls learn about snowshoes, about what they could do, and where they could go with them." She was already in her 50s when she grabbed the opportunity to learn snowshoe lacing from Marlene Patch, a Tubbs lacer for 32 years. She is also a snowshoe detective who has diagramed patterns of antique snowshoes sent to her from all over the country for relacing. She long ago lost track of how many snowshoes she has laced.

If you too are gripped by the romance and aesthetics of traditional wooden shoes, sign up for a long weekend of snowshoe making and snowshoeing at the Gunflint Lodge in northern Minnesota. You'll come back with a pickerel snowshoe that you yourself wove. John Silliman, the lodge's naturalist and snowshoe maker, teaches guests how to lace snowshoes from a kit that contains a pre-drilled bentwood frame. After a group has made their snowshoes, which takes a day and a half or so, Silliman leads them on a snowshoe hike. Moose abound in the area, and one might also spot a fox, wolf, coyote, pine marten, snowshoe hare, or, with extraordinary good fortune, an elusive lynx. If northern Minnesota is not in your travel plans, you can order a snowshoeing kit to use at home. (See Resources on page 129.)

As noted earlier, modern snowshoes date back to the 1970s and the development of the first aluminum-frame models in the Pacific Northwest. Smaller than even the most compact wood frame shoe, but with an assertively upturned toe and a solid, synthetic decking material in place of lacing or webbing, this early type of modern snowshoe (also called a **Western** snowshoe) was substantially lighter, more maneuverable, and more durable than wood ones. Western snowshoes gathered many fans, first among the mountaineering community and eventually among the early recreationist adapters, who viewed snowshoeing as an end unto itself rather than as an approach tool for winter mountaineering. Some purists continue to prefer old-style wooden models but the great majority of snowshoers today use modern aluminum-frame or molded plastic snowshoes.

Anatomy of a snowshoe

To accomplish the function for which they were designed, snowshoes today must meet four basic performance criteria. First, they must provide flotation on the snow, so that the wearer does not sink far below the surface. Second, while they are attached to the boot, they must rotate underfoot, allowing the boot to pivot so that the snowshoer can walk naturally and adjust to changes in slope pitch and other terrain variations. Third, snowshoes must provide traction both on uphills and downhills. Finally, snowshoes must be comfortable, both in terms of weight and shape, to minimize fatigue and maximize the natural stride over snow. Even the most primitive snowshoes basically met the first two criteria. The third was partially met with later wood-frame snowshoes because the webbing itself offered some traction, but the fourth was only possible with the appearance of modern snowshoes.

The snowshoe's frame is its skeleton, and like a crustacean, that skeleton is on the outside. Traditional snowshoes have been made of many types of wood, but ash has long ranked as the favorite. Steamed and bent into the shapes described on pages 17–18, the strong frame remains functional even under trying conditions. Within it is the soft part, a web of intricately laced strips of rawhide wrapped around the wood to support the snowshoer's weight on the snow. Crossbars built into the tip and tail sections stabilize the frame, keep it from warping, and alleviate some of the strain on the rawhide or other lacing. Both the crossbars and the lacing provide decent traction on all snow conditions except ice. The rawhide webbing or lacing was later coated with shellac to protect it. A Minnesota snowshoe maker named Charles Iverson began replacing rawhide with a synthetic rubber called neoprene, and by the 1960s, other makers did so too. In time, neoprene was replaced by other, lighter weight synthetics. Whatever the material, the lacing in a rounded wooden frame resembles a tennis racquet, but with a hole in the webbing to allow the foot to flex and the boot toe to pass through — still a key feature in snowshoe designs. The tennis-racquet image dies hard — and in French, snowshoes are actually called *raquettes*. In a

Dennis the Menace comic strip, Dennis ties racquets onto his friend Joey's feet and reassures him that his parents "don't play tennis when there's snow on the ground." Popular image notwithstanding, most snowshoes today are made of a tubular aluminum frame with synthetic fabric decking to keep the user near the surface of the snow, crampons underneath for traction and stability, and an easy-to-use binding to hold the snowshoe firmly to the boot while allowing the foot to move. A smaller shoe made of these contemporary materials provides users with better performance and greater stability than a larger one of traditional design.

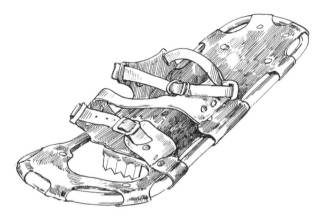

aluminum-frame snowshoe

Over time, there have been about as many kinds of traditional bindings as there have been traditional snowshoes. The most basic binding is nothing more than two straps, one over the toe or instep and one that looped behind the heel to hold the boot onto the snowshoe, but even more advanced bindings are simple. A woven nylon strap might zigzag across the foot to hold it snugly. There might be two fore-foot straps and one heel strap. Ratchets rather than slide buckles might be used to tighten the binding. Or there might be a sort of spat with a shoelace-type closure. Bindings are now integrated into snowshoe design, and every one, from simple woven-nylon straps and plastic buckles to microadjustable ratchet models, have made snowshoeing easier. Some snowshoe/binding combinations have added features, such as a rigid plate that fits under the entire boot sole to provide additional stability or built-in heel lifts (an MSR [Mountain Safety Research] innovation called the "Televator") for climbing steep slopes. Mountaineers and backcountry snowboarders who often climb steep slopes particularly appreciate such features. Step-in bindings, which are standard for Alpine and cross-country skiing, could be the next frontier in binding design. In the late '90s, Bill Prater and Andy Davis offered a step-in binding for crampon-compatible mountaineering boots. And in the early 21st century, snowshoe maker TSL and boot maker Lowa came out with an integrated boot/binding combination. Redfeather has a binding that easily ("automatically," the company avers) adjusts to both the front and back of the boot.

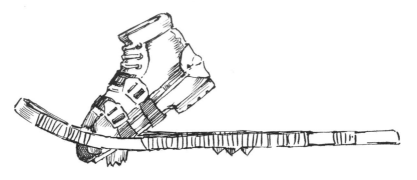

foot moving through plane of snowshoe

Just as in the old days of simple straps, what makes these newer snowshoe/binding combinations functional and what is still important in modern bindings is a system that enables the foot to move freely and naturally while walking. To allow such free heel use, there must be a hole in the decking, and bindings have to pivot around something. That "something" was the toe cord, originally made of leather, and later neoprene (or, under the Sherpa design, a rotating steel rod), under the ball of the foot, which allowed the heel to lift and the foot to flex. Today's binding is hinged around a rod (or other material flexible enough to pivot) that serves the same purpose as the old toe cord. That pivot point,

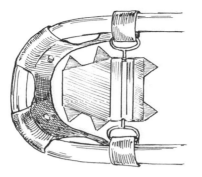

crampon (claw) detail

where the binding attaches to the decking, is located under the ball of the foot. It enables you to walk naturally and comfortably and also to climb uphill.

The amount that particular bindings pivot varies among models, but basically, there are now two types. The "full rotation" design allows the greatest range of motion for the snowshoe, which can drop vertically (that is, up to 90 degrees) from the upraised foot. Because powder sloughs off the back of the snowshoe with each step, it is especially popular for snowshoeing up steep slopes and in deep, loose snow. With a "fixed rotation" or "fixed hinge" design, the tail drop is limited to about 45 degrees. This keeps the snowshoe deck closer to the boot sole, offers more control, and is less tiring than a full rotation model. It is popular for trail use on packed snow. Rotation also adds control, allows "tracking" or steering in deep snow, and enables you to position your foot to kick steps into the snow on steep slopes. Remember that toe hole? It is still part of the snowshoe design, whether using a free rotation or fixed pivot system. It's there so that the boot toe can move through the plane of the snowshoe and the foot can flex fully during the stride, maximizing the functionality of the pivot system.

Modern snowshoes also allow for the incorporation of traction devices, on both aluminum and plastic models. Variously called claws, cleats, crampons, or talons, these metal gripping devices underfoot prove practical on uphill climbs and provide reliable traction even on hardpack. Most snowshoes feature one set of traction devices under the forefoot and another set under the tail of the snowshoe. They are effective in preventing backsliding while climbing, but they can make it difficult to back up, even on flat terrain. Taken as a complete snowshoe/binding/traction unit, modern snowshoes weigh about a third less than the old wooden models.

Even as aluminum-frame snowshoes became standard, a second late 20th-century trend was the development of injection-molded plastic models. Mountain Safety Research (MSR) brought out the Denali series of performance molded-plastic snowshoes, but in general in North America, plastic was less popular than aluminum-frame models.

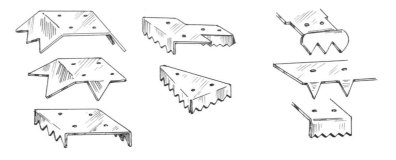

styles of crampons: front claw   *heel cleats*

Still, the use of this type of material paved the way for snowshoes that are lightweight, easy on the budget, and available in eye-catching colors. Here, plastic snowshoes are most popular for children (designs that resemble animal paws are particularly cute), casual snowshoe walks on mellow terrain, and even as part of the emergency supplies and survival gear that well-prepared north-country drivers carry in their vehicles. Yeti makes a simple survival snowshoe of webbed plastic just for such purposes. For backcountry use, beefier models come with clip-on or slide-on extenders for additional flotation in deep, soft snow. In Europe, heavy-duty plastic is extremely popular, with both one-piece designs and models with plastic frames and lacing available.

The Big Transition

"I was a snowshoeing virgin until about 11 years old," recalls John Woodbury, who grew up in Anchorage, where he is now a writer, photographer, editor, and publisher of *Coast Magazine* as well as an accomplished outdoorsman. "Before I knew how to walk like a duck while staying afloat upon Alaska powder, I was content to posthole through snowdrifts in search of ptarmigan, snowshoe hares, and solace. It wasn't until I and two chums, Neil Rome and Chris Curgus, got serious about stalking our state bird that we discovered it was a much fairer chase when both predator and prey wore walking aids. The ptarmigan had their tufted, feather-covered feet, and we had our snowshoes.

"My first set of snowshoes, a Christmas gift out of an L. L. Bean catalog, were of the bearpaw variety. The round, catgut snow slippers were a dream. Small enough to weave through alder patches, yet large enough to give a sniffly-nosed youth some loft atop even the most dainty snowpack. The problems were that the bearpaws were almost useless when it came to traversing a slope, and the binders were beyond frustrating. On one lengthy three-day trek into the Chugach State Park, a half-million acre playground behind my childhood home, my snowshoes became cruel shoes. While the lacing and shoes were of quality construction, the binders were cheap. The second day into the trek, the metal buckle snapped, forcing me to create a makeshift binding out of a headlamp elastic band just to get back to civilization.

"Eventually, even that rough-hewn binder failed, so I was forced to slip my boots under the toe hole on the shoe. I hiked this way for seven miles, but did manage to make it out of the woods. My near-frozen toes took some time to heal, and my enthusiasm for snowshoeing went frigid too. Only lately have I rediscovered the beauty of snowshoeing. The snowshoes and binders have improved, as has my attitude toward the sport."

My own epiphany about the value of modern shoes came, surprisingly, on a hot weekend in June in the Colorado high country — quite a contrast to John's experience. My husband and I were planning a late-spring weekend of hiking near Aspen when a magazine editor phoned and said, "We want to run a story about snowshoeing in Colorado. I understand you write about skiing. Can you write about snowshoeing?" Of course, I said, knowing that I could still find snow at high elevations at that time of year, the perfect opportunity for some basic research. With borrowed state-of-the-art snowshoes strapped to our packs, we set off on the Cathedral Lake Trail that very weekend. You cannot imagine how foolish we felt on a shorts-and-T-shirt day — until we neared the lake and began meeting earlier birds who were already on their way down. "You were smart to bring snowshoes," we were told several times. "There's still a lot of snow up there, and it's soft."

The 11,886-foot Alpine lake is set in a basin sheltered by mountains, where snow packs in starting with fall's first flakes, piles up deep, and lingers long. Even in late June, snowmelt had not bared the cirque in which the lake nestles. First, we encountered patches of snow. Then, sun-softened snow swales left over from mid-winter drifts. Finally, as we approached the lake, cobalt blue from recently melted snow, we started crossing a seamless cover of deep corn-mush snow. While other hikers were post-holing, we waltzed across the snow surface on our snowshoes and felt quite pleased with ourselves. Any snowshoes would have been better than no snowshoes, but the modern metal-frame ones dramatized the contrast between my first miserable experience and my second satisfying one.

The Revolution Continues

Just as wooden snowshoes evolved, so have the newer metal and plastic ones, with choices of size, material, frame shape, binding design, and other components that were undreamed of a couple of decades ago. By the end of the 1980s, the shift in design and materials was well underway, providing a launching platform for the rocket-like rise of snowshoeing in the 1990s and beyond. New compact shapes enable the snowshoer to stand normally and stride naturally without the awkward and exhausting straddle walk of old. Also, cute fun-themed designs for

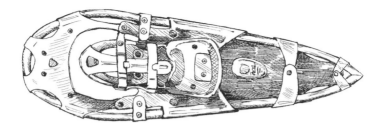

tapered snowshoe

children and special models for women are now standard in many manufacturers' product lines. For women, snowshoes have narrower, tapered tails and bindings to hold smaller, narrower boots.

San Francisco-based Atlas was the first snowshoe manufacturer to offer spring-loaded bindings, while Crescent Moon came up with radically tapered tails and what it calls its "foot-glove" binding, featuring an injection-molded stirrup, single-pull forefoot adjustment, and a ratcheted heel strap. Designed to distribute tension throughout the binding system, regardless of boot size, this binding adjusts from women's size 5 to men's size 14. A couple of manufacturers, Atlas and PowderWings, make collapsible snowshoes that come apart to easily fit into a small fanny pack or stuff sack for easy carrying over snow-free terrain and for assembly on the spot when they are to be used. Yupi Skishoe is a shortski/snowshoe hybrid that resembles a snowshoe but has a sliding surface for downhill sliding, and Verts makes a small, inexpensive toe-forward snowshoe especially designed for climbing.

Materials are increasingly high-tech. MSR's model uses a tough snow-shedding co-polymer (polyethylene and polypropylene) that is stable in subfreezing temperatures and hardened-steel crampons and traction bars that reportedly outlast aluminum five times to one and are powder-coated to prevent snow from sticking. Tubbs now uses ultra-rugged titanium for the crampons on some high-end models, and to keep the snow from clumping underfoot, has added a melt plate and a split-front crampon. Innovations have accelerated as snowshoeing has become more popular. In Europe, where plastic prevails, some snowshoes even make a fashion statement. Chanel boutiques in the French

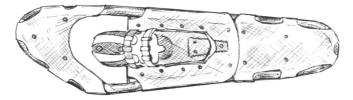

asymmetrical snowshoe

Alps carry molded-plastic snowshoes custom-made in white with red and white bindings. They are stylish indeed, yet they remind me a bit of the Tenth Mountain Division's big old beavertails painted white for camouflage. Perhaps Chanel designers, too, thought that white snowshoes would give users the ethereal look of floating on the snow. Arguably the most important user-friendly adaptation is an asymmetrical shape to the snowshoe shape. These snowshoes themselves, not just the bindings, come in mirror images, right and left, like street shoes or ski boots. Some people find that walking is simply more comfortable with asymmetrical designs, with different tapers at the tails. Women, with wider hips and greater tendency to be knock-kneed rather than bowlegged, and runners, who really need to *not* step on their own snowshoes, like this design. By contrast, symmetrical models differ only in the placement of the binding. The buckle is supposed to go on the outside of the foot, but less flexible people often find it easier to fasten the binding when the buckle is on the inside.

Which Shoe for You?

One thing about modern snowshoes that should simplify your buying decision is that in terms of quality, you *can't* really go wrong. By and large, modern snowshoes are all good. In fact, snowshoe makers' generous warranties indicate how confident manufacturers are of the quality and durability of their products. Other than availability in your area, the variables to consider are the appropriate size for your weight and planned use, and the price you are willing to pay. Today's snowshoes come in such different shapes and ranges of size that you should easily find one that works for you. Attend a demo day where you can try out various brands and models of snowshoes, or rent a few times to test different ones.

The right snowshoe size is a function both of your weight — not on the bathroom scale when you've just gotten out of the shower, but when you are dressed in winter clothing and carrying a loaded pack — and the snow conditions under which you will be using them. Many snowshoe manufacturers print catalogs with extensive model descriptions, including the snowshoes' dimensions, weight, material specifications, and often a chart for recommended sizes. This information is often posted on their Web sites as well. Some specialty outdoor gear retailers also have assembled this information into a buying guide. Of course, sales personnel at such stores can also make recommendations. Adult snowshoes come in three size ranges. Snowshoes that are 7 or 8 by 21 inches are best for mountain or trail running on packed snow. If you weigh 150 pounds or less with winter clothing and a pack, you'll be looking at models that are about 8 by 21 to 8 by 25 inches for women or 9 by 25 for men. These medium-size, multipurpose snowshoes can be considered the sport's golden mean, suitable for most adults to use for recreational day hiking on packed snow, broken trail, settled snow, or fresh powder over a firm base. Some adults weighing between 150 and 175 pounds prefer slightly larger snowshoes, measuring 9 by 25 inches for women and 9 by 30 inches for men, especially if they hike in soft snow. Those weighing between 175 and 200 pounds might be looking at a 9- by 34-inch snowshoe, and people weighing in at 200 pounds or more and winter backpackers carrying heavy loads should consider snowshoes that measure out to a substantial 10 by 25 to 36 inches. All other things being equal, select a slightly larger snowshoe than these weight guidelines if you expect to be doing a lot of hiking off-trail or in light powder. Specialized snowshoes complete the spectrum on each end with small children's snowshoes (6 to 7 by 15 to 17 inches) on the low-performance, moderately-priced end and heavy-duty models designed for mountaineering expeditions or aggressive running on the high-performance, high-priced end.

While it is clear that, all other things being equal, a small shoe isn't enough for deep powder (you will sink) and a large shoe is more than most people need on packed snow, experts say that another factor (in balancing maximum snowshoe performance with minimum snowshoer fatigue) is the snowshoes' weight. I have heard various comparisons, ranging from "1 pound on the foot is like 3 pounds on the back" to "1 pound on the foot is like more than 5 pounds on the back." Running snowshoes usually weigh under 3 pounds per pair. Midsize, multi-purpose snowshoes weigh between 3 and 4.5 pounds per pair. Heavy-duty backcountry behemoths can weigh 5 pounds or more. Just do the math. The bottom line is, don't buy a bigger snowshoe than you'll need for the conditions you'll encounter most of the time.

Price considerations are linked to size and types of material. If you are a new snowshoer, aren't a heavyweight, don't plan on carrying a big pack, and are likely to stay in local parks, well-used and packed trails, or such controlled venues as Nordic centers or Alpine ski areas, an economical model with a fixed-rotation toe cord and non-technical plastic decking will do just fine. In fact, if that describes you, you might consider a snowshoe kit (value snowshoes, poles, and an instructional video or a tote bag), made by such reputable manufactures as Tubbs and Atlas. If you weigh more, carry a hefty pack or perhaps a toddler in a carrier, or explore the more remote backcountry, you'll want to invest in more expensive snowshoes made of heavier-duty material.

What, you might ask, is the bottom line? Suggested retail prices for aluminum-frame snowshoes with integrated bindings at full retail generally range from $100 for low-end models all the way to $400 for super-high-performace racing shoes. For most adults, recreational snowshoe design options in the low-to-middle price range are more than adequate. End-of-season specials, closeouts, and sales of rental snowshoes are among the ways to cut the cost even more. Still, considering that some people use their snowshoes year after year after year, and that (except for trail fees to access Nordic areas, lift-accessed trails at Alpine areas, and the occasional public-lands use fee) snowshoeing is usually free, the equipment represents a minor investment for major winter pleasure.

I wrote the first snowshoe-specific trail guide to Colorado, and I'm often asked which snowshoes I use to explore trails in the Rocky Mountains. I'm neither a heavyweight nor an endurance athlete nor a winter backpacker . . . nor, in truth, a gearhead. I've hiked many miles alternating between two moderately priced, mid-size models by popular manufacturers. Both have fixed-rotation bindings, and though I often snowshoe in soft Rockies powder, I haven't really lusted for a full-rotation shoe. Eventually, though, I plan to get women's snowshoes, mainly because I'm getting tired of tightening unisex bindings to my size five boot. In addition to my own two pairs, I've also occasionally tried many other brands, and I can't really claim a strong preference for any one over the others. They might be different in the way they look, adjust, and feel, but by and large all are just dandy in the way they perform for me. Still, I do have a favorite pair of snowshoes. I particularly treasure a pair of Tubbs wooden snowshoes that have never been set on snow, a pair hand-laced by Joan Scribner-Lemieux (who, as I explained, has kept the art of snowshoe lacing alive in Vermont) and inscribed to me on the wooden frame. I often wonder what will happen to that legacy once K2 winds down its Stowe operation and moves at least some of its production of modern snowshoes to China.

Another aspect of the sport's versatility, as it relates to equipment, is the variety of suitable footwear. Some manufacturers offer snowshoe-specific boots, which are insulated, waterproof, and designed to slide into snowshoe bindings, but these aren't really necessary. I've snowshoed for years on Salomon Winter-X boots, heavy-duty, insulated winter hikers that are no longer in the product line. Just as you select snowshoes to match your activity and terrain, choose well-fitting footwear that matches your snowshoeing needs as well. For hiking on packed trails, waterproof leather or synthetic hiking boots work well if you are mostly concerned with support, or waterproof, insulated boots like those made by Sorel are better if warmth is more important to you than support. Mountaineers on approach routes use their hard-shell plastic mountaineering boots, while runners favor lightweight running shoes, often with neoprene socks or toe covers to keep their feet warm. Wool or wool-blend hiking socks, perhaps with wicking liners, will help keep your feet dry and warm. Gore-Tex or nylon gaiters will keep snow from seeping into your boot tops.

Snowshoewear

There is not, as yet, a type of clothing called snowshoewear in the same sense as skiwear, swimwear, or tenniswear. If you have been a winter hiker or live in the north country, you probably know all you need to about dressing for snowshoeing, because it's a lot like dressing for cross-country skiing, winter hiking, or perhaps just trekking to the grocery store. You have a winter wardrobe for the outdoors filled with high-tech longjohns that wick perspiration from your body yet retain warmth, synthetic pile, called fleece, jackets and vests for insulation, and waterproof and breathable outer garments designed to combat rigorous winter weather. Increasingly popular are soft-shell outer garments, which combine comfort, stretchability, breathability, and water-resistance. These materials, which are fabricated into pants and jackets, work for all but the most frigid or wettest conditions. Whatever the fabric and insulation or style of garment, everything has zippers so that you can vent when you are warm and zip up when you begin to feel chilled. You will already own such winter active-sports accessories as headgear (a fleece hat in temperate climates and a wool or insulated balaclava where it's really cold) and waterproof, windproof ski gloves or mittens, or a combination of windproof shells and glove liners for cold days and lighter fleece gloves or even just glove liners on mild ones.

When layering, the clothing progression is simple, really. First, you put on a polypropylene or other wicking base layer next to your skin to keep your torso warm and dry. Then you add a mid-layer of Polartec or other synthetic fleece on your upper body, perhaps an insulated vest if needed on those near-zero days. You top it all off with a waterproof, wind-resistant yet breathable outer layer of Gore-Tex or other synthetic. On relatively mild days, it might be a single-layer anorak or light training jacket. A hat that can be pulled down over your ears is essential. Fleece, wool, or a lined helmet design of insulated fabric are popular choices. When it's really cold and blustery, or you will be hiking at high elevations, you'll probably want a heavy-duty backcountry jacket with a high collar and a built-in hood. You keep your lower body comfortable by wearing fleece, stretch thermals, or winter running tights with or without windproof pants, depending on the weather.

Snowshoeing Accessories

Poles are an optional extra for some snowshoers and must-haves for others. Count me among the latter. I like poles to maintain a rhythm while hiking uphill, for added stability on downhills or sidehills, for additional traction if needed, and to knock snow off my snowshoe claws if I've hiked across moist snow, perhaps from a spring or creek, or late in the season when snow tends to stick to the metal. Anyone heading up steep hills can use poles to add more power to each step. The best designs for snowshoeing are adjustable or telescoping backcountry ski poles with generous baskets. Shorten both poles on uphills, lengthen them on downhills, and make one longer and one shorter for extended sidehill traverses.

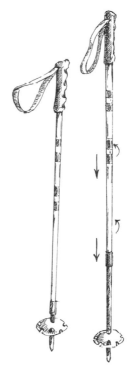

Gaiters are useful for cold, windy days. I always have with me a stretch fleece neck gaiter for cold windy days and the aforementioned over-gaiters to cover boot tops and lower legs. A product called Wristies are stretchy Polartec tubes that slide over your wrists to keep that vulnerable spot between your jacket cuffs and the tops of your gloves warm. It's especially useful for long-limbed snowshoers,

adjustable poles

whose jacket sleeves never seem quite long enough. Sunscreen and sunglasses or even ski goggles when it's really cold or windy help shield your eyes from UV rays, unpleasant glare, and drying out from the wind. They also protect your eyes from whippy branches when you are snowshoeing through the brush.

Because you are wearing layers that you might take off or put on as the day warms or cools, as the wind picks up or dies down, or as your body temperature changes with the effort of snowshoeing, you will need a day pack to hold extras.

Snowshoers tuck different things into their day packs, but here's what I always take for a backcountry day hike:

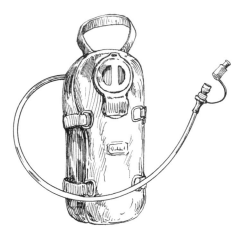

backpack hydration set-up

• Insulated hydration pack filled with water. I use a Camelbak with a neoprene sleeve covering the drinking tube and heavy rubber cover for the bite valve to keep the water from freezing. Sipping frequently will also help prevent freeze-up.

• A Thermos of hot soup or hot tea and a peanut butter sandwich on whole-grain bread, which comprise my favorite winter trail lunch, plus a couple of energy bars and/or trail mix for snacks.

- Extra socks, gloves, hat, and shoelaces.
- Cotton neckerchief.
- Swiss Army Knife or other multi-purpose utility knife.
- Compass and waterproof, tear-resistant map. (I favor Trails Illustrated maps for the backcountry and always pick up a trail map at a Nordic center; see "Stepping Out," chapter four.) A photocopy of the trail description of your hiking route from a reliable guidebook is a nice extra too.
- Single-use hand- and foot-warmers. Activate by taking them out of the package and shaking them. Use according to directions on the outer wrapper, but do not unwrap until you need them.
- For emergencies, a lightweight Mylar "space blanket," small first-aid kit including adhesive blister pads and Band-Aids, waterproof matches, small flashlight, and whistle — none of which, thankfully, I've ever used.
- Small book that identifies animal tracks in the snow.

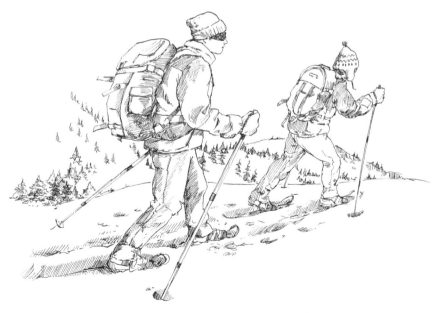

snowshoer (rear) with backpack; snowshoer (front) with day pack

What I carry in winter is not all that different from what I carry in summer on a comparable hike. When snowshoeing at a Nordic center, especially on a clement day, I might just take a small waist pack with water, a snack, and a trail map. And, because I am a writer who considers every snowshoe hike to be a research opportunity, I always have a notebook in my pocket, a pen stuck up my sleeve to prevent it from freezing, and a water-resistant point-and-shoot camera tucked into my jacket. When you begin to appreciate the beauty of the winter world, you might want to take a camera, too, to record your snowshoeing adventures.

three

The Winter World

The pleasures and perils of the snowy season

SnowSports Industries America launched an image campaign called "Winter Feels Good." When I heard about it, I could only wonder: What took them so long? No one has ever needed to tell me that winter feels good, but it seems that this seasonal truth is not self-evident to everyone. I'm one of those people who enjoy the progression of the seasons and treasure each one's special pleasures. I love the rejuvenation, fresh growth, and promise of spring; the intensity and abundance of summer that fulfill spring's promise, and the sparkling days and brilliant foliage of autumn that represent a last burst of summer heat and energy. In late fall, after the leaves have fallen, the earth seems to fold in on itself, heralding winter to complete the cycle.

Here in Colorado where I live year-round, summer days are blazingly beautiful, but winter is never far away. I've been snowed on every month of the year, not only during winter storms but occasionally also during high-elevation summer hikes when snow squalls roll in. I live just at the base of the Rockies at 5,400 feet, and since I moved to Colorado in 1988, the earliest measurable snow in my yard fell on September 5 and the last snow of the season fell on May 11. At this elevation, fall and spring snows disappear quickly, and even in winter, they melt to the ground on the frequent balmy days to be replaced by another blanket of white down during the next storm. But in the mountains, winter is not an ephemeral season. Come fall, temperatures drop, and wetlands crust up and then freeze solid enough to walk over. Snow settles on the dark green boughs of pine, spruce, and fir, and frosts the tawny tundra. High lakes glaze over, first just skimmed with a crinkly crust over overnight ice, then soon frozen deep. When snow piles on the glassy surfaces, snowshoeing routes cross them as if they were solid earth. Before long, the landscape is completely white, and it stays that way until spring snowmelt. As winter deepens, storms can come in ferociously, brutal blizzards that are incentives to stay indoors. Or snow can fall calmly, with cloud-light flakes drifting from the sky that are invitations to go outside. But whether it comes cruelly or kindly, snow grips the high country, covering the mountains and the valleys, the forests and the open meadows, the ski trails and the golf courses. And it seems like it's just waiting for us to explore it and enjoy it.

Few activities equal and none exceeds the sheer satisfaction and joy of a snowshoe hike. On many a winter morning, I saddle up my Subaru and drive to a trailhead, strap on my snowshoes, and head out into that winter world, preferably with my husband or a friend for companionship and security. But snowshoeing directly from my front door has added the satisfying dimension of instant gratification to the sport. The first time I did it was soon after I got my first pair of modern snowshoes — not borrowed, not rented, but *mine* — and I was antsy to try them out. Soon after the snowshoes arrived, so did a storm that lasted from Friday afternoon until early Sunday morning. The snow lay deep on branches, rooftops, and cars, muffling the city of Boulder under 8 or 9 inches. On Sunday morning, day broke tranquilly. There was no wind and no traffic, so I got up with the sun, dressed quickly, strapped on my snowshoes, grabbed my poles, and started walking.

My destination was the nearby trailhead for Sanitas Valley, one of a cluster of popular local hikes. A wide route lying between Hogback Ridge and Mount Sanitas, it was originally the road to a long-defunct quarry on the flank of Mount Sanitas. The road is just a mile long with a steady, sometimes steep incline. It was a quick hike that my husband and I (and seemingly half of our neighbors) had done countless times before work on summer mornings. How different it was in winter, on snowshoes! Only two sets of tracks preceded mine, and I chose to break my own trail along the edge. I loved making my way through the soft drifts, intentionally kicking up a snowshoe full of light powder and watching my own little mini-snowfall drift back to the ground. The seamless snow on the slopes on either side of the trail had been broken here and there by deer and smaller animals. I puffed up the steep parts, cruised on the gentler ones, and soon I stood on the small plateau at the top of the trail. From there, I gazed eastward across the city and to the plains beyond and to the rising sun that blazed bright — and I looked back down at the trail, where traffic had picked up considerably. Having savored the best of the snow and the solitude, I started down. As I descended, a procession of snowshoers, skiers, walkers, joggers, and dogs was on its way up. The rapidly rising sun began softening the snow on the south-facing trail, degrading the snow surface. I had gotten the best of the snow during a quiet part of the day. With snowshoes, you can often do the same.

John Woodbury of Anchorage, Alaska, whom you met in chapter two, doesn't even have to go as far as I do to get off the street and onto a trail. The self-described "sniffly-nosed teenager" who first explored the backcountry on wood bearpaws eventually bought his boyhood home near Chugach State Park and now lives on five acres.

"I nipped alder bushes around my property line and set a snowshoe trail for snowy winters," he reports. Since his boyhood, he says, "The shoes and binders have improved, as has my attitude toward the sport. The route at Compound W, which is what I call my house, meanders to nowhere in particular, but it provides me with stellar vistas of the front range of the Chugach and, most importantly, a much-needed 15-minute-a-lap break from my computer and all that deadline stress that constantly haunts a freelance writer and photographer. Instead of bearpaws, I've graduated to a pair of MSR Denali Ascent snowshoes, a high-tech, molded plastic shoe with aggressive spikes and claws for mountain snowshoeing. The bindings consist of rubber straps that take one hand to buckle. They always stay snug and right where they are supposed to be. While I compromise a bit on loft with the stubby Ascents, I gain much in stability when traversing sidehills or rugged terrain. If the snow is really deep and granulated, however, I heft the old bearpaws off the living room wall, where my girlfriend — much to my dismay — 'retired' them. I consider it blasphemous to retire perfectly good equipment before its time, but also recognize compromise is sometimes necessary to maintain a peaceful household. I wrap the shoddy binders around my boots and trudge into winter's majesty, and a few feet closer to my childhood."

I consider my Sanitas Valley hike to have been a perfect little snowshoe excursion on a well-traveled, hazard-free route that was close to home, with quiet, solitude, and pleasant weather. John Woodbury finds circuits around his backyard to be a head-clearer when he needs one. Many hometown snowshoe walks can have the same effect, whether in a park, on a recreational path, or a snow-covered street. But when you are going into the outback, you need to be weather and snow savvy in order to get the most out of your experience and stay safe.

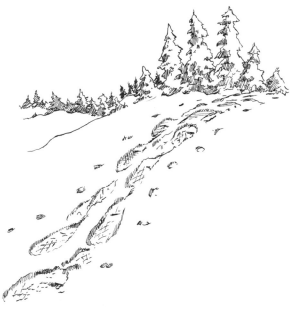

snowshoe tracks in snow

Snow Story

People have snowshoed on sand dunes and probably other nontraditional surfaces too, but by and large, the common denominator for snowshoeing is, of course, snow. The North American snowbelt stretches across the northern tier of the lower 48 states, Canada, and Alaska and at high elevations down the spines of the Sierra Nevada, the Rockies, and, to an extent, the Appalachians. That's a lot of real estate covered with snow for three to five months of the year, and much of it is accessible on snowshoes.

Snow forms when atmospheric moisture adheres to small solid particulates and builds into a crystal. In the coldest climates (at the poles and at the highest elevations) snow falls as small pellets. In such relatively temperate regions as the northern United States and southern Canada, the flakes that fall are fat — moist on the coastal ranges and near the Great Lakes and drier inland.

North America's weather follows distinct patterns. Hurricanes and nor'easters aside, most of our weather systems form over the Pacific Ocean. Moisture-laden air then moves eastward over the continental land mass and butts up against the Cascades and Sierra Nevada, dropping snow on the mountains. The snow clouds dry out as they pass over the interior deserts of the Northwest and the Great Basin, but then dump generous accumulations of normally light snow on the Rockies. Snow also falls on and blows across the northern plains. The Great Lakes create their own auxiliary weather systems, known as "lake-effect storms," which unleash abundant snowfalls on the upper Midwest and Northeast. These regions benefit from those storms too, but the warming effect of the Atlantic Ocean also makes near-coast areas vulnerable to more rain, ice rain, sleet, and midwinter thaw cycles than other parts of the north country. And Canada, rightly called "the great white north" by the fictitious Mackenzie brothers of *Second City Television* fame, is snow central, with virtually a coast-to-coast blanket of white. Temperature, humidity, storm intensity, snowpack depth, wind conditions, thaw-freeze cycle, slope pitch, and slope exposure are among the variables that determine the snow conditions you will encounter along the trail during any hike anywhere on the continent, and these can change from day to day or hour to hour along the same route.

Winter Life

At first glance, the winter world might look lifeless. Especially during a storm, when nothing seems to be moving except branches of wind-whipped conifers, we are tempted to think of a stark and empty black-and-white world from which most bird species have migrated and other animals have escaped by hibernating. But a closer look reveals winter to be full of life and activity, and in the calm that follows each storm, we may encounter animals, and we will certainly see signs of their presence.

Animals deal with snow and cold in one of three ways. They may migrate long or short distances to avoid the most extreme winter in their habitat. Caribou herds of the far north migrate long distances, while elk and deer migrate more locally. Animals may hibernate, a state also called "winter sleep," living off stored fat until spring. Finally, they may adapt to winter, growing thick coats of fur, developing large paws to stay on top of the snow, or turning white as camouflage against predators. Birds either fly south or adapt.

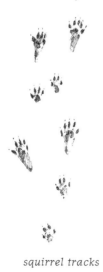

squirrel tracks

Tracks of rabbits, squirrels, weasels, snowshoe hare, and chipmunks form arcs, loops, and straightaways. Where there is prey, there are predators, such as coyote, fox, wildcat, and wolf, which are all active in winter, and you will also see their tracks. I particularly liked an analogy I heard from Lina Polvi, a Swedish-born naturalist with the Aspen Center for Environmental Studies, who called these tracks "the fourth dimension." She described tracks as representing the dimension of time measured since the last snowfall. She views new snow as a blank sheet of paper, and animal tracks are like marks

fox tracks

on the paper that can be read by the observant passerby. If they are crisp and look the way they do in a track-identification book, it means the animal passed by recently, certainly since the last snowfall. When the edges get fuzzy and the shapes are harder to discern, the animal passed some time ago. And when new snow fills old tracks, it is like tearing off the marked-up paper and starting with a fresh sheet. While evidence of small animals abounds in winter, it is somehow more thrilling to find traces of bigger species. Deer, elk, moose, and other big game forage in their winter feeding grounds, and evidence of these large ungulates abounds along backcountry snowshoe routes, with fresh hoof prints and scat. The South Elbert Trail, a four-wheel drive road to a summer trailhead for Colorado's highest peak, morphs into a splendid route that passes through a major elk wintering ground. Even when the herd is not in sight, hoof-packed snow reveals that the animals are somewhere nearby.

Anyone can be a wildlife detective in the snow. It's easy to see where the little critters scampered from tree to tree, for food is easier to find under branches than in the deep snow. Birds' claw prints are etched into the snow where they light for a seed, a nut, or perhaps a crumb dropped by a snowshoer or skier. A scattering of scales under a conifer means that a squirrel has dissected pinecones, eaten the pine nuts, and dropped the scales under the tree. Where there is prey, predator tracks are likely to be found. Coyotes, foxes, and cats leave their tracks across the snowy landscape. If a few days have passed since the last storm, and a trail has been well used by humans, many animals (especially large, heavier ones that sink into soft snow) understandably save energy by moving along a human-tracked path. Seeing animal tracks is fun, and I carry

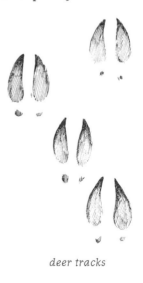

deer tracks

a track guide in my winter pack, much as I carry a wildflower book in summer. In truth, the only ones I'm pretty good at identifying are rabbit (one set of large paw prints and one set of small ones), pine squirrel (tracks resembling the Batman symbol), and porcupine (a furrow "plowed" into the snow by its low-slung body).

Still, I always get more of a thrill out of seeing the animal itself than trying to figure out what made the tracks. It was hard to miss, or misidentify, the moose browsing in Jim Creek across the valley from Colorado's Winter Park Ski Area, the herd of elk occupying a clearing and spilling onto the trail at Alberta's Jasper Park Lodge, or the deer skittishly running across the low-elevation trail in Rocky Mountain National Park. Again in Colorado, I've watched a porcupine cross a trail right in front of me at Beaver Creek, and at Steamboat, I spotted another perched high in a pine tree, nibbling on bark.

Two animal encounters stand out in my memory, and both involve bison. The first time, I was staying at Spring Creek Resort, a mesa-top spread near Jackson, Wyoming. I explored the rolling ranchland in the valley below that had been turned into the resort's equestrian center in the summer and Nordic center in the winter. Some elk and a couple of deer were browsing near the entrance to the corral. Either they had been habituated to the hay set out for the livestock, or the old ranch had been built along a traditional wildlife migration route and the herds had never changed their patterns. I saw a porcupine's furrowed track leading to a tree where its lumpy form could be seen. I had also been told that bison hang out in willow thickets not far off the trail, and indeed, I saw a couple of large, dark masses that might have been hunkered-down bison — or perhaps merely rocks or dense brush piles.

After rambling around the Nordic trails, I decided to snowshoe up to the resort via a back route instead of returning via the van shuttle. The day was achingly beautiful, with blue skies, brilliant, slanting sunshine that made the big red barn stand out in the snowy landscape, and just a few fluffy clouds hanging on the high peaks of the Teton range. I turned around for once last look at the valley just before the trail wrapped around the mesa, and there, on the hillside just a few hundred feet behind me, were three big bison. One was lying in the snow, one was standing up staring at me, and one appeared to be eating a tree. It was one of those literally breathtaking moments. I was greatly thrilled but a tad uneasy, because I was alone and outnumbered as well as out-weighed by the shaggy trio.

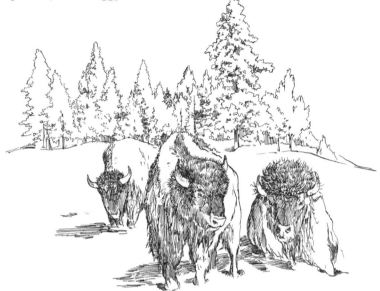

bison in snow

Several years later, some friends and I were snowshoeing to the Lone Star Geyser in Yellowstone National Park. Though less pre-dictable by the clock than Old Faithful, it provides more bang for your snowshoeing buck because each eruption lasts 15 minutes or longer. The geyser is an easy two-and-a-half-mile hike along a wide, flat trail along the Fire Hole River. We rounded another bend in another trail and found another bison, not 50 feet off the trail. He — or maybe she, I certainly couldn't tell — was standing in belly-deep snow near the river, slowly swinging its massive head back and forth to push the snow aside and reach edible vegetation. The sound it made was a muffled snort, and the attention he paid to us was none at all, even when we stopped to gape, gaze, and photograph. I felt no discomfort because I was with other snowshoers, and there was, after all, just one bison.

Such thrilling encounters with large animals are more likely in winter than any other time of year. Animals tend to winter where there are more food sources — in sheltered valleys, in semi-open areas where forest meets open meadow, in riparian areas — and they conserve their energy by staying in place unless they feel threatened. Speaking of threats, people with little backcountry experience wonder about predators. Foxes, coyotes, and other North American canine predators do not usually go after anything as large as adult humans. Nor do bobcats, mountain lions, or other feline predators.

As thrilling and as exciting as it is to share large animals' habitat, caution always pays off, both for the creatures' sakes and for yours. Remember, wild lands are not zoos. Especially in places like Yellowstone, Banff, or Jasper National Parks, where wildlife is habituated to human intrusion, it is important to remain cautious, wary, and respectful. Do not approach animals for photography or just to get a closer look. A zoom lens is better than a close encounter. Remember that wild animals are unpredictable, especially if they feel threatened or are startled. If you encounter bison, moose, or elk — especially those who might be pregnant and still be protective of their young from the last birth cycle — wait for them to move away from your route. If they don't move, it is up to you to do so, and carefully. Detour around them, giving them wide berth; 25 yards is generally considered a safe and sensible minimum distance. Keep in mind that you cannot outrun them, especially in deep snow. If the park or any natural area permits dogs, keep yours leashed to prevent it from chasing or harassing wildlife.

In protecting themselves against what they perceive as a human threat, some animals can expend so much energy that they themselves are traumatized. When a species is rare, a grave threat perceived by a single animal is magnified even more and can impact a herd's viability. In Canada's Jasper National Park, for example, wardens (the Canadian term for "rangers") especially warn visitors to the Maligne Valley to watch out for mountain caribou, which live here year round. Winter is a particularly critical time for these animals, who expend a great deal of energy searching for food in the valley's deep snows. The females, who are pregnant in winter, must maintain their strength: The success of their pregnancy depends on it, and those calves mean a lot to a species on the brink. These caribou see extremely well and are disturbed by the sight of people or dogs, even from a considerable distance. Visitors can stress them without even knowing it. Dependence on humans for food also endangers animals, so it should go without saying that you should never feed large or small animals in the wild. When they become dependent on handouts from humans, they lose their ability to survive on their own.

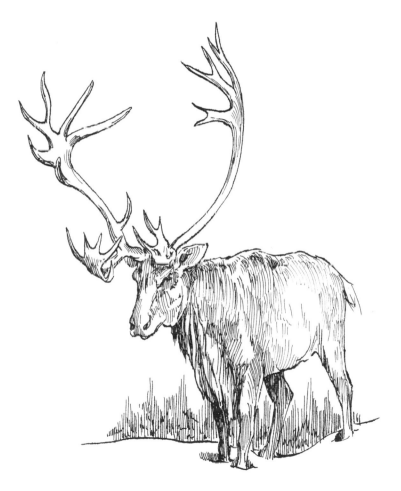

caribou in snow

Some of my most pleasurable and enlightening snowshoeing experiences have been in the company of a naturalist guide who understands animal behavior, can identify plants in their slumber state, and is conversant with geology, geography, snow morphology, and other aspects of the natural world. Some of these tours have been conducted by park rangers, others by naturalists connected with local conservation organizations or resorts, and still others by licensed commercial guide/outfitters — all serious outdoor folk with a deep love for their territory and knowledge to match. I've learned something from every tour I've taken.

Naturalist tours can take some unexpected twists, as I found out in Les Arcs, France. I joined a group following in the wake of Bernard Bruley, an *accompagnateur en montagne* (loosely translated as one who accompanies guests in the mountains) as opposed to a *guide de montagne* (as hard-core licensed climbing and mountaineering guides are called). This bespeckled, puckish man was improbably costumed in a Davy Crockett-like buckskin outfit, coonskin cap, mountaineering boots, and plastic snowshoes. Instead of a musket over his shoulder, an old 35-millimeter rangefinder camera was slung around his neck. He was firing off a volley of mixed fashion messages that I hadn't thought a Frenchman could possibly achieve.

Europeans might not think it strange to start a nature walk by clumping across a paved parking lot on the backside of a modernistic slopeside village development, with views of dumpsters, cigarette butt-infested snowpiles, and laundry airing on surrounding *balcons,* but to Americans, it seemed like an inauspicious start for a wilderness experience and, in fact, it brought such a humorous element to snowshoeing that a few of us were giggling hard at the sight we presented. But soon, we were proceeding at a good clip down a snow-covered path through what would be considered a small forested area by North American standards; in France, it was designated as a *zone de protection de la nature.* A little protection goes a long way in the French Alps. The trees were dense and varied, and the trail was litter-free. Bernard chatted about the fauna and the creatures that inhabit the woods and the surrounding mountains. He spoke about deer and rabbits in the forest zone, the *chamois,* a small goat-like antelope that lives on the rocky ledges of the Vanoise National Park and other places in the high Alps, and the vegetation on which these animals survive.

He spoke of the wild mushrooms that would appear in the summer, as well as the wild herbs that grow under the trees and in the clearings. I was particularly taken with his discourse about "the charming pussy willows" along the way. How "French" to find so perfect an adjective for this species. And how "French," too, that our snowshoe walk ended at a tiny farming hamlet called Le Planay, now designated as a "gastronomic village." We unstrapped our snowshoes at the door of an old, old house, and entered what had become a small rustic restaurant. Out came the bottled water, the wine, the exquisite soup, the platters of Savoyard sausages and cheeses, the baskets of toothsome bread. Never have I taken a snowshoe walk that began with less promise and ended with a more congenial and civilized finale.

Another special night-snowshoeing experience took place in the Vallée de Joux, the heart of Switzerland's watch-making industry. A group of us snowshoed from the tranquil village of Le Sentier in the fading afternoon light. We skirted farms and entered the forest, our way illuminated by moonlight. Following local guides, we wound the long way through the thickening trees to an old woodsman's cabin that was the last word in rustic simplicity, with a woodstove, lanterns for lighting, and heavy tables flanked by wooden benches for furnishings. First came the mineral water and wine, of course. Then came platters of steaming *croûtes aux morilles,* roasted bread topped with succulent mushrooms that are found in spring just after snowmelt, dried, and then reconstituted the following winter. A local sausage of ground pork and chopped cabbage and potatoes in leek purée comprised the entrée, and a divine apple tart served well as dessert. It wasn't easy, bending down over full tummies to rebuckle our snowshoes for the return to Le Sentier along a wide road that was, fortunately, mostly downhill.

Not every beguiling snowshoe experience has to be in such a distant or exotic locale. Kurt Repanshek, an avid and experienced Utah hiker and outdoorsman, has learned to appreciate fleeting wildlife encounters as a bonus to a snowshoe hike. "The subdivision I live in, about eight miles north of Park City proper, has 600 acres of open space in the form of a sprawling east-to-west mountainside covered by scrub oak. A couple of years ago, the Park City-based Mountain Trails Foundation cut hiking/biking/snowshoeing trails across this hillside, and while snowshoeing there, I've seen mule deer, elk, moose, and snowshoe hares," he reported. "One evening, I spooked a snowshoe hare, which was pretty cool. He was a big guy. I've also seen ermine at the White Pine Touring Center in Park City. While on a snowshoe hike up Lamb's Canyon, about 15 miles east of Salt Lake City, I spied what most likely was a golden eagle. On the return to the trailhead, I startled a grouse. On another hike, deep snow forced me to park about a mile or so from the start of the trail. Still, it was a nice hike to the trailhead, as the road parallels a creek that was busy with ducks. Now all I need to do is figure out exactly what kind of ducks!"

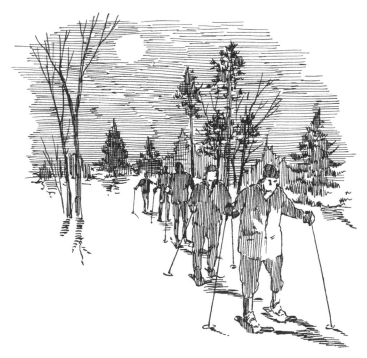

snowshoers on a moonlit hike

With or without rich feasts at the end of the trail, moonlight snow-shoe hikes can be the most memorable hikes of the season. Moonlight snowshoe hikes take on a special glow that always makes me think of the line from *The Night Before Christmas:* "The moon on the breast of the new-fallen snow gave the lustre of mid-day to objects below." One of my favorite full-moon routes is the one to the Lefthand Reservoir just outside the Indian Peaks Wilderness. This wide, snow-covered road, less than an hour's drive from my home, climbs 580 feet in 1.8 miles and culminates in a capacious valley. The frozen reservoir is one flat white sheet startlingly brilliant in the strong moonlight, bordered by a ruffle of dark conifers. Beyond are the flanks of Niwot Ridge and such Indian Peaks as Arikaree, Kiowa, Apache, Shoshoni, and Navajo, gleaming like silver against the ink-black sky.

Perhaps you too will find a favorite night-snowshoeing destination. Sign up for an organized moonlight tour, or create your own. On a clear night just before or at full moon, dress especially warmly and find a wide trail or meadow and start walking. You'll be astonished how bright the scene can be and how quickly your eyes adjust to the unaccustomed light source. A trail is easy to follow out and back or in a loop. If you select a meadow, you'll want to make sure that the snow is fresh enough for you to return easily by retracing your own steps and that you hug the edges and follow a fenceline or a wall to create a loop. All the better if you are familiar with the way from a daylight hike because things do look different at night, no matter how bright the moonlight. But don't just look down at the trail. Be sure to look up at the night sky, sprinkled with stars.

Cautions and Precautions

Though the whole idea is to enjoy snowshoeing's pleasures, it's wise to be aware of potential winter perils, especially when exploring the backcountry. Legitimate winter threats are by and large preventable by preparing for weather changes with adequate clothing, backcountry navigation and route-finding skills, and an awareness of avalanche danger in slide-prone areas. A friend with considerable outdoor knowl-edge (but who asked that his name not be in this book because "I don't want people to know how stupid I was") recalls a scary snowshoeing excursion in the mid-'70s. He and a friend rented a pair of Alaskan snowshoes for what they intended to be a short winter backpacking trip in the Sierra Nevada. Strong and cocky from their recently completed Army experience, they were equipped, he says, with "youth, strength, enthusiasm, and 'reading experience'" rather than real experience in the winter backcountry. They set off on a beautiful day with a summer tent, lightweight sleeping bags, and inadequate clothing for the rough win-ter conditions that they did not anticipate.

"We hiked over the west ridge of Castle Peak and the west ridge of Basin Peak," he recalls as if it were a recent misadventure. "We camped in a grove of trees, but during the night, the wind came up. In the morn-ing, we struck camp and started to head out. We could get up to the ridge but got so windchilled that we couldn't proceed, so we headed back to our campsite. We tried several times and were beaten back by the wind each time. The frustrating thing is that from the high point, we could see the Sierra Club's Peter Grubb Hut with smoke coming out of the chimney. We were tired from the cold and from our repeated ascents up the ridge. We just couldn't get ourselves and our big packs to warmth, shelter, and safety. After two mornings, we knew we were in a bad spot and had to go. We left everything but the clothing on our backs and went back to the trailhead as fast as we could."

He wouldn't make a mistake like that again, and with today's equip-ment and clothing, neither should you. The greatest hazards in the winter backcountry are hypothermia and dehydration, with frostbite running a close third. A short, local snowshoe walk like my Sanitas Valley experience or one at a Nordic ski center, dude ranch, or other controlled venue doesn't normally require preparations for such contin-gencies. But for backcountry trips, it is wise to be prepared for a change in the weather, an injury, or other unforeseen circumstances. To maxi-mize upside pleasure, minimize the downside risk when planning a snowshoeing excursion. This book is not meant to be a winter emergency or first-aid text (many such books are available, as are courses for serious backcountry adventurers), but even the most casual snowshoer and winter explorer should know some basics. These worst-case scenarios are meant to caution you, not to scare you.

Hypothermia is becoming chilled . . . very chilled. It occurs when the body is unable to maintain normal internal temperature because more heat from the core is lost than the circulatory system is able to provide. At best, when the condition is mild and of short duration and body heat is restored to normal levels through physical activity, heavier clothing or blankets, or even through the help of sunshine, it is uncomfortable and slightly disorienting. At worst, hypothermia can be fatal. The air does not need to be extremely cold for hypothermia to set in. Not to be an alarmist, but rather a realist, I would remind you that when someone is said to have frozen to death, the cause was severe hypothermia. Preventing it is a balancing game. You must keep the body from losing so much heat that the core temperature drops. Wearing properly protective clothing, staying physically active, and drinking enough water are preventive measures.

The early signs of mild hypothermia are collectively nicknamed "the umbles." The first signs are that a person begins to stumble, mumble, fumble, and grumble. The cure is warming the core as quickly as possible. It may be as simple as putting on an extra layer of clothing and returning to a warm building or a heated vehicle as quickly as possible. The first sign of severe hypothermia is uncontrollable shivering, often accompanied by genuine disorientation. This condition is a real medical emergency and is not to be trifled with. It is, fortunately, rather unlikely in a recreational snowshoeing situation under most conditions. When you snowshoe for pleasure and exercise, you are not about to go out in the most extreme conditions without adequate clothing and other preparation . . . are you?

Frostbite, which is not the same as hypothermia, affects the surface of the skin and the extremities, rather than the core. It starts as tingling, called frost nip, then degenerates into numbing, and finally to an absence of feeling. With frost nip, there is still some feeling in the affected parts. It is easily dealt with. Inserting disposable heat packs into boots or gloves, adding dry glove liners, or changing to dry socks will often cure it. When frostbite sets in, the affected extremity becomes numb. The skin surface turns white, as the body tries to protect its core by concentrating blood where it is needed for survival, rather than near the skin. If the skin is still soft, frostbite is considered mild. When the skin becomes hard and extremely pale, the condition is serious and again is a medical emergency. Frostbite can be caused by direct exposure of the skin to raw cold and can be beefed up by wind or inadequate protection, especially at the fingertips and toes.

The best cure, of course, is prevention. Here are some basic winter practices to keep you comfortable and safe:

Take (and wear) enough protective clothing. Remember the layering principle outlined in chapter two (page 32). Start with a base layer next to the skin, add an insulating mid-layer, and top it all with a wind-

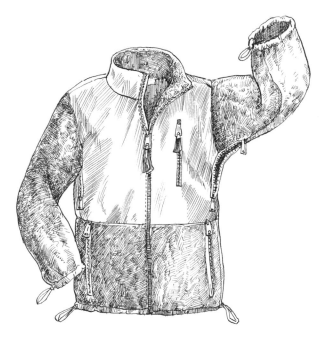

outer layer jacket

proof, water-repellent, yet breathable outer layer. Performance outdoor clothing will have a drawstring at the waist and perhaps one at the hem of the jacket to trap body heat inside the shell, as well as underarm zippers, called "pit zips," that you can open if you need to vent body heat during exertion. At the very least, make sure that your insulating layer and outer jacket are high-collared. Some people like wool or fleece scarves, but I also prefer a stretch fleece neck gaiter so that body heat does not escape at the neck. If it is warm and sunny, or you are working hard while snowshoeing uphill, you can always unzip or shed a layer and put clothing in your pack until you need it again. If you might be out in wet falling snow or even sleet (marginal, drippy precipitation that snowshoers in the Cascade and coast ranges anticipate and those along the Atlantic coast occasionally experience), be extra-sure that your outer layer is very rainproof. And top your winter tights or fleece with rainproof shell pants to keep your lower body warm, and a hat to prevent heat loss from your head.

Stay dry. It is critical that the base layer wicks moisture from the body and transmits it out through the mid- and outer-layer garments. Remember that chilled perspiration sucks body heat as it evaporates, which can lead to hypothermia. As a corollary, remember that the most effective winter undergarments are today's synthetics. Don't even think about wearing old-fashioned cotton longjohns. In fact, don't consider cotton clothing at all in the winter backcountry. (Jeans are a real no-no, except on a short, close-to-the-trailhead hike on a nice day.) Wet cotton chills. By contrast, wool, though not currently in high favor for backcountry layering, retains warmth even when wet. And, as I noted above, if you live in an area where snow is very wet or where it tends to sleet, be sure that your clothing is rainproof, too. The flip side of dressing warmly enough is that it is possible to get overheated. Again, remember that perspiration that accumulates on your body rather than being wicked away will cool you off when temperatures drop. That's why a wicking layer and the venting functions of the mid- and outer layers are so important.

Wear a hat. Up to 40 percent of body heat can be lost when a person is bareheaded. If wool has a place anywhere in the winter backcountry wardrobe, it is for headgear. A thick wool-knit hat with earflaps is cheap added insurance against hypothermia. By contrast, if you have been working hard and are getting overheated, taking your hat off for a few minutes, or changing to a lighter one, is a quick way to cool off.

Remain hydrated. Hot tea, kept in a Thermos, counts toward your water intake, but it is important also to take and drink water steadily through your hike. In fact, drink more than you think you'll need. An active adult requires as much as two quarts of water a day to remain properly hydrated. You might tend not to feel as thirsty in winter as you do in summer, and it's easy to forget that thirst lags behind the early stages of dehydration. Simply breathing in the cold winter air, perspiring as you hike, or being overdressed can all cause a fluid loss in the body, but drinking enough maintains the balance. It is easier than ever to stay hydrated (which means drinking enough water to help prevent hypothermia) with modern and convenient hydration systems (see chapter two, page 34).

In winter, you probably need to take simple measures to keep your water supply from freezing up. Fill your water bottle or hydration pack with tepid or even warm water. It will cool off soon enough. Some people fill up with water that is shot with an electrolyte solution (sports drink), lemon or orange juice, or a little schnapps or other alcohol to lower the freezing point. I stick my insulated Camelbak in my pack, but I know other people who prefer to tuck their hydration systems inside their jackets. Any system can choke with ice if even a small section of the tube is exposed to the cold air, so be sure that the neoprene sleeve snugs up against the insulated bite valve. If you prefer a conventional water bottle in a holster, put it in upside down, because the top of the water freezes first, so ice will form at the bottom of your bottle.

One of the clues that you are drinking enough water is the need to urinate, which can be a challenge in the winter backcountry. Men have it easy here. Step off the trail, step behind a tree or rock, unzip, do what you have to, kick some fresh white snow over the yellow snow, zip up, and you are done. For women on the trail it's all a little more complicated: find a discreet off-trail spot — behind a bigger tree, a boulder, or a clump of bushes, stick your poles in the snow on either side for added stability if you need them, unzip, unbutton, or whatever, and squat in a wide-legged stance. If you choose to use toilet paper or tissue paper, either burn it (and pile snow over the ashes) or take it out with you in a zip baggie. I prefer just to scoop a handful of snow. It's cold for a moment, but the minute you pull your layers up again, you'll warm up fast. Pull up your pants, zip up, kick fresh snow on the yellow snow. You can diminish the number of times you have to go through this exercise by using a pit toilet or outhouse at the trailhead, whether you need to go or not, before you start hiking. Some Nordic centers provide occasional trailside facilities — a welcome convenience.

Keep your fingers and toes toasty. Fingertips and toes are especially vulnerable to frostbite, more so in women than in men. Warm socks and warm handwear provide the first line of defense. For the feet, heavy hiking socks are suitable under waterproof boots, with wool or wool-blend recommended. I also carry an extra pair of dry socks and have changed in mid-trail if my socks somehow got wet. I wear Thinsulate-lined winter hiking boots. Select boots that are snug and supportive when worn with your socks of choice, but not so tight as to constrict circulation to the toes. Heavy-duty mountaineering boots and winter Mukluks are even warmer. Some people add wool-felt or newer-generation Thinsulate insoles. And remember gaiters keep snow from entering your boot tops. For the hands, invest in good-quality gloves, a glove system consisting of an inner insulating glove and an outer shell for wind protection and to keep your hands dry when you have touched the snow, or try mittens for extra warmth. Add thin glove liners if needed. I am also a great fan of inexpensive, chemically activated handwarmers and toe warmers, available at outdoor stores, ski retailers, and north-country convenience stores. And when you're snowshoeing with poles, don't grasp them in such a death grip that you cut off blood flow to your fingers.

Protect your face. Exposed areas are particularly vulnerable to frostbite when it's very cold, more so with the addition of windchill. Make sure your hat covers your earlobes, and if it doesn't, add a headband of fleece or wool. A turned-up jacket collar and a neck gaiter pulled up over your mouth and nose can ward off frostbite, but for severe cold (the kind that I frankly don't want to be out in), a face mask of neoprene or wool offers additional protection. Goggles, rather than sunglasses, cover more of your face. With a hat or headband pulled down and a neck gaiter or mask pulled up to the goggle frame, you can minimize the risk of frostbite even in severe conditions.

Use sunscreen. Protect your face from sun as well as from cold. Sunscreen is not just for the beach. Snow reflects sun rays and the thinner air at high elevations allows more UV rays through. Sunburn and collateral skin damage are easily preventable.

Don't snowshoe alone. Go with a group or at least one other person — or even with a faithful dog of a breed or mix that can handle oversnow travel. A human companion can alert you to the telltale white patches that indicate frostbite, and when it comes to route-finding, which I'll discuss in the next chapter, two or more heads and two or more sets of eyes on the map and the compass are better than one.

High-Mountain Cautions

Some environments pose threats not found in others. A basic precaution on sunny days is, of course, **sun protection,** and the higher the elevation at which you are snowshoeing, the more conscientious you need to be about it. For your eyes, wear quality sunglasses with ultraviolet ray filtration. Wraparound models are a good idea, or go for goggles, which are best in extreme weather such as deep cold, wind, or snowstorm. Sunscreen is a must on exposed skin. SPF 15 is the minimum for most complexions, and SPF 30 is reasonable if you are fair-skinned. Lip balm that contains UV protection will prevent burned lips and even prevent them from becoming chapped. Sunscreen and lip balm should be reapplied while you are out. Skin cancer is no joke, but even if that were not a potential problem, sunburn isn't fun. **Windburn** is sunburn's cousin. A facemask, scarf, or neck gaiter pulled over your chin, nose, and cheeks can prevent it when the wind starts howling.

Everyone breathes harder when exercising at elevations that are substantially higher than where they live, but for sea-level dwellers snowshoeing in the mountains, **altitude sickness** can be a problem. It is unrelated to age or physical condition and can strike some people at elevations as low as 5,000 feet. Most lowlanders will feel some effects at 8,000 or 9,000 feet, and people who are prone to it will begin feeling ill then. A dull headache, thirst, and perhaps some nausea or even mild disorientation are early symptoms, which some people interpret as a cold, jet lag, or even a hangover. Preventive measures include taking it easy the first couple of days, drinking plenty of water, avoiding alcohol and cutting down on caffeine, and, if possible, spending a night or two at a relatively lower elevation before heading for the real high country. Symptoms usually disappear in a few days, when the body has acclimatized, but if you are visiting, that can take a big chunk out of the average trip.

Another concern is **avalanche** potential in the West, where mountains that reach to and above the treeline and hefty snowfall are facts of winter life. This ferocious force of nature can pose a real threat in the backcountry, claiming a couple of dozen lives in the United States and Canada every year — mostly backcountry skiers, snowboarders, and snowmobilers. Skiers and snowboarders yearn for above-the-treeline steeps, and snowmobilers, with their range and ability to set off slides, comprise the greatest number of casualties. There really is no reason for most snowshoers to venture into the riskiest terrain, though snowshoes' versatility sometimes leads people into temptation and delivers them into a hazard zone. As one Gunnison National Forest ranger once said to me, "No trail is without any avalanche hazard." And that is only slight hyperbole in some places. The bottom line is that recreational snowshoers on even the most benign Western routes should have rudimentary avalanche knowledge, acquired by taking an avalanche awareness course, going on a few guided tours — and paying attention to guides and drawing on their experience when on a tour. Check avalanche reports, issued statewide or regionally, before venturing into the backcountry. Finally, if in doubt, turn back rather than risk a hazardous area.

Eighty percent of avalanches occur during or just after major snowstorms, but that also means that 20 percent happen at other times. Skiers or snowshoers crossing an unstable slope and snowmobilers cutting across an open area can trigger avalanches. The safest part of the snow season is generally in late winter or spring when the snow has settled and stabilized — except when it isn't. Open slopes angled at more than 30 degrees are the most likely to slide. Slides can occur when the snow is unstable (including in the early season when cover is thin) or when freeze-thaw-snowfall cycles have caused instability between snow layers. Check local outdoor organizations or sporting-goods stores for reasonably-priced avalanche awareness programs if you live in a region with known hazards.

In this chapter, I've outlined some of the potential problems, but please go back and read the section above called "Winter Life," because while the problems are, as I stated, potential, the wonders are real. So is the fitness dividend you'll reap every time you go out on snowshoes.

four

Stepping Out

Easy introductions to the snowshoeing world

There's a joke that getting started in snowshoeing is a 12-step program. The punch line is, "Take 12 steps and you're a snowshoer." There is scarcely such a thing as a snowshoeing lesson, as it is understood in most sports, but rather just quick tips to shortcut the already minimal learning curve. In fact, I'll wager that there are few outdoor activities that are as simple as snowshoeing. Just about all you need to do is to *decide* to do it. Snowshoeing involves little more than putting one foot in front of the other, and remember that you already know how to walk. It might take a few minutes to get used to having gear on your feet that flops up and down with each step. Walk a few paces on flat terrain, and you're a snowshoer — and if your ambitions never extend beyond wintry strolls on mild terrain close to home, you won't need more than that. In fact, the biggest challenge to some newcomers to the sport is figuring out how to put the snowshoes on so that they stay on; with modern gear, even that is simple. It isn't much more complicated than getting into a car and fastening the seatbelt, and someone at the rental or retail shop will even show you how to do it before you take the snowshoes out the door.

Back in the early '70s, when cross-country skiing experienced a big boom, adherents used to say, "If you can walk, you can ski." For some people, that was indeed true, but for others, it was a misleading claim.

Cross-country skiing required a certain confidence to slide and stride on long, skinny boards. Many beginners, especially those who had never downhill skied, felt that cross-country skis were tippy, found that sliding even on a gentle downslope could be scary, and had problems moving uphill. Not so with snowshoeing, which is as simple as walking. The snowshoes act as steady platforms, generally preventing even the uncoordinated from falling; the crampons on the bottom of the snowshoes grip while ascending; and the snowshoes are not designed to slide on downhills. With this in mind, all you need to do is strap your snowshoes firmly onto your feet and start walking on a flat, snow-covered area, such as a meadow, a park, or even your unshoveled driveway.

On packed rather than loose powder snow, the feeling of snowshoeing is very similar to walking on bare ground. You will need to decide whether you want to snowshoe with poles. If you are or ever have been a skier, poles will feel comfortable for you. If skiing has never been part of your life, think of poles as nothing more than an extension of your arms. If you do use poles (which more and more snowshoers are doing), plant your right pole as you step forward on your left foot and your left pole as you step forward on your right. As you walk and move "through" your pole plant, release the back pole as you tip the front pole into the snow. If you choose not to use poles, walk as you would on dry land with your arms swinging naturally: left foot/right arm and right foot/left arm. If your snowshoes are of proper size, this normal gait is no problem at all. Notice that I wrote "walking," not "shuffling." With crampons on the bottom of your snowshoes, you should pick up your feet just a little, not a lot, something akin to wading in shallow water. As you lift each foot forward to take a step, you will notice that the snowshoe tip rises and the tail drags lightly behind you. That is as it should be, as the result of the snowshoe's built-in pivot system. As you step down on the next foot, that snowshoe flattens against the ground and the crampons dig into the snow.

When you look at snowshoes, you might think that you will be treading on your own big feet with every step. With old wooden snowshoes, it used to be a problem for some people, but no more. Traditional snowshoes, which were generally wider than modern metal-frame designs, caused many snowshoers to adjust their walking patterns to avoid stepping on the other snowshoe, which in turn contributed to hip pain. Today's narrower designs, whose flotation comes from a smaller surface of solid decking rather than a greater surface area of open-weave lacing, avoid that problem, and such refinements as tapered, asymmetrical, and special women's models avoid it still more.

After you've walked on the flat, look for a little hill to walk up and down a few times. As you are ascending, keep your weight over your feet without leaning forward. Notice how the crampons dig into the snow. Their grip prevents backsliding. When descending, again keep your weight over your feet, without leaning backward. If the slope is gentle, walking downhill feels virtually the same as walking on the flat, but if the slope steepens a little, get into the habit of keeping your knees flexed as you descend. This puts more definite pressure on the crampons to give a firmer bite in the snow. You don't have to worry about the crampons catching in the snow, because they are angled to release with each step as you walk either up or down. The flip side of crampon design is that backing up on snowshoes is difficult or, for some people, downright impossible.

So how do you change direction? The easiest way, of course, is just to walk in a big circle, but that only works if you have enough room to do so. To make a U-turn on a trail or other confined area, you'll need to do a step turn. It's more complicated to describe than to accomplish. Hold your poles comfortably far from your body so that your snowshoes have room to turn within them. You can perform a step turn in either direction, but for simplicity here, I'm describing a left turn: With your weight on your right foot, rotate your left foot 90 degrees, taking care not to bang the tail of the left snowshoe into your right ankle or to step on your right snowshoe. Next, place your left foot firmly on the snow. Then, pivot your right foot parallel to it, while rotating your body to remain square with your feet. Again, put your weight on your right foot, and repeat the maneuver. You will then have turned around completely. If you are not flexible enough for a 90-degree turn with each step, take three or four smaller-angle steps to complete the maneuver.

It's easy to get hooked on snowshoeing. Dave Felkley did. Once a high-profile district manager in the high-pressure automotive world (think Nissan USA and Mercedes-Benz), Felkley changed his life. He

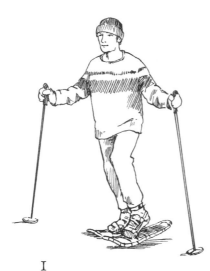

I

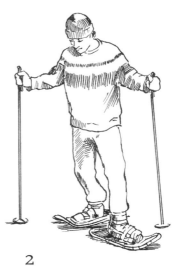

2

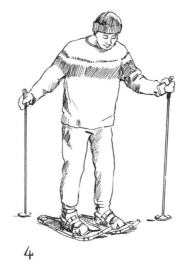

3 4

sequence of step turn

likes to say that he "traded his wingtips for hiking boots, and the Mercedes for mountain trails." He now lives at 8,500 feet in the laid-back hamlet of Nederland, Colorado. When he's out on the snow-shoeing trail, his answering machine explains that he is out under "the big blue dome." His business, BIGfoot Snowshoe Tours, is lower-key than anything in the automotive world, and when he's not guiding clients or snowshoeing with friends, he likes to frolic outside with one of his three grandchildren. Come to think of it, out there, he's as much of a kid as they are.

The Next Steps

Experienced hikers, who generally comport themselves safely in the out-doors, pick up snowshoeing in an eye blink. They adjust easily to terrain and slope variations, know how to read a map, and can set right out on a fairly ambitious snowshoe hike. But if your trail experience is limited or you aren't sure of how you will handle the additional weight of heavy boots plus snowshoes as you walk, start sensibly. Sign up for an easy snowshoe outing with a sports shop, a guide, a park ranger, or a local club that offers outdoor activities. If you're not into group excursions, find a friend to join you on your first snowshoeing venture. Pick a fairly flat route so that you can get accustomed to the sensation of snowshoes. You will soon feel the subtle rhythm of the snowshoes pivoting under your feet, and you will feel the security and stability that snowshoes provide. Look around at the beauty of the winter world, and you too will soon be hooked.

Beyond the basics, the snowshoes themselves present little limitation on where you can go or what you can do. Even at the beginning of your snowshoeing career, a bit of experimentation on varied terrain that includes both uphills and downhills and different snow conditions will extend your range considerably. You can amble, stride, jog, or even run on these big feet. Eventually, you can use them to race over snow, embark on serious winter hikes, or backpack to a winter camp-site (see chapter five for more information on campsites). In short, snowshoeing can take you where you want to go. You might want to go on a snow-covered trail in a nearby state, provincial, or county park, national forest, or even national park. There is a lot to be said for selecting a route that you are familiar with from summer hiking, though the winter backcountry looks a lot different.

After a few modest outings, you'll have an idea of your stamina, especially in challenging weather or in unpacked, untracked snow. As soon as your ambitions and desires extend beyond the easy and safe snowshoeing context of a guided group or a controlled environment, you need to think about boosting your skills, both in terms of a few slightly more advanced snowshoeing moves and also in terms of route-finding and general backcountry skills and knowledge. You might have gotten your snowshoeing legs under you by walking up and down gentle hills, but as you get further into the sport (unless you hike on pancake-flat terrain in, say, central Illinois), you will eventually be tackling steeper terrain that requires some modification to the straight-up, straight-down walking of mild slopes. You will find poles helpful for all of the following moves.

Steep ascents. As the pitch steepens, shorten each ascending step and think about consciously shifting your weight to the toes of your boots as you ascend to minimize fatigue and maximize traction. When the slope gets *really* steep, conditions dictate how to handle it. If the surface is loose, unpacked snow or sun-crust over powder, aggressively kick the front of each snowshoe into the snow and then firmly put your weight on it to pack down a snowshoe-size platform with each step. You will effectively be kicking steps into snow, so that your foot is close to horizontal each time. Be sure that your stance is solid before you lift your foot out and begin the next, higher kick-step. If the snow is packed down firmly or even icy, just march straight uphill, digging your crampons into the hard surface with every step you take. If the snowshoes function as they should, but you are still huffing and puffing uncomfortably during a steep ascent, make switchbacks up the slope (see page 68).

Traversing across a slope. Keeping your weight on the uphill side of each snowshoe, press the uphill side of the frame into the loose snow with each step. Quality snowshoes have some lateral torsion, so that you won't be stressing your knee and ankle joints as you cross a slope. As with the kick-step, the idea is to keep your snowshoes as near to a horizontal position as possible. Since crampons are not intended to prevent side-slipping, you will find this technique to be the most secure. Additionally, if your traverse is long and you are using adjustable poles, you might wish to make the uphill pole shorter than the downhill pole, which will make it easier to keep your body weight square over your feet.

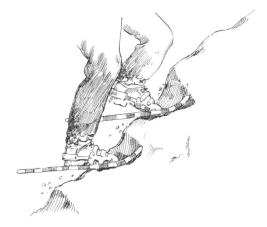

kick-step in steep ascent

Steep descents. Keep your weight balanced over your heels to enable the heel crampon to grip. The idea is to have your weight over your heels in a centered position, but not to press your weight onto the tails of your snowshoes. In powder, you can *glissade,* a French word meaning "slide" or "glide." When glissading, you allow the heel crampon to release to essentially ride the snowshoe downhill a little way with each step. With your body weight squarely over your feet, flex your knees lightly and begin lightly running downhill. You will slide a little with each step before the combination of your body weight and the crampons slow you. Inertia and gravity help you glissade, which is more fun than you can imagine.

Switchbacking up a hill. If you are following a marked trail, your route is predetermined, but if you are bushwhacking and the going gets steep, you can make your own route by serpentining up the hill, creating your own energy-saving switchback route. Angle up the slope in one direction, then turn to angle up the other way. If you are using short snowshoes, a turn of this type is easy. If you are using long shoes and perhaps carrying a big pack, you might have to do kick-turns to change direction.

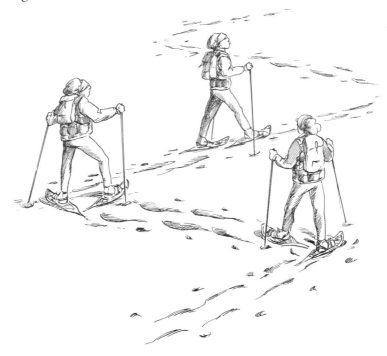

switchbacking

Handling deep snow. Moving through loose, unpacked snow requires more energy and is therefore more tiring than snowshoeing on a packed trail. Remember that your snowshoes will not keep you afloat on the surface of the snow, but they will prevent you from sinking in too deeply. The snowshoe's pivot point allows it to rotate underfoot so that loose snow will slide off the back, but in the deep stuff, you don't have to take total advantage of that feature. As you move along, you will conserve energy if you submarine your snowshoes under the surface of the snow at their natural level rather than trying to lift the snowshoes out with every step. Powder days provide another reason not to snowshoe alone, because another way to conserve energy is to take turns breaking trail. The lead snowshoer moves along, plowing a furrow through the loose snow and packing it down somewhat underfoot. The second snowshoer has it easier, and by the time three or four people have followed, the original track is a packed-down route, making following still easier. Some people like to lead and break trail until they are tired, then drop to the end of the queue and let others take their turns in the lead. Other groups establish a rotation, either by keeping track of time or by counting steps.

Snowshoeing in spring. Spring brings warm sunshine, mild weather, and soft snow. It is a time to enjoy snowshoeing picnics and the balmy whiff of spring. It is also a time when snow can get very soft, especially on sun-struck slopes. Two cautions are necessary. First, stay on packed trails to avoid sinking into deep, soft snow. Second, be informed about avalanche danger in slide zones, because spring is the season when slab avalanches are more likely to occur. In short, spring is really a season to stick to packed, marked trails — and break out a picnic to celebrate the most benign part of the snowshoeing season.

Falling and getting up. Despite the stability of your snowshoes, it is inevitable that you will, someday, fall. Everyone does, and it's no big deal. The snow usually acts as a cushion, and injuries are rare. There are several ways to get up, and poles are always useful. If you are carrying a heavy backpack, you might want to unstrap it before hoisting yourself and it out of the snow. Sit on one hip with your snowshoes parallel to each other. If there is a firm base, grip your poles, simply push the tips into the snow, and use them and your leg and upper body muscles to get upright. In deep snow, cross your poles into an X, hold them in one hand where they cross, and use them to help push yourself upright. Of course, a hand-to-wrist grip and a tug from a companion work well, too.

Smart Moves for Smooth Starts

When people without a lot of hiking or outdoor experience ask me about the most hassle-free way to begin snowshoeing, I always suggest that they join a group. The leader or guide is there to scope out the terrain, help with any equipment problems, answer questions, and point out interesting things along the way. If you know that you are capable of maintaining a brisk hiking pace over distance, investigate snowshoe tours run by a local outdoor group, such as the Sierra Club, the Appalachian Mountain Club, or a similar organization where you live. The outings hustle along aggressively, but a group excursion geared for beginners always moves at a more moderate pace that is ideal for building skills and confidence.

I once joined two couples from the Carolinas on a snowshoe tour out along the ridge on the backside of Aspen Mountain, led by Aspen Center for Environmental Studies naturalist Rebecca Lemburg Weiss. Both men and one of the women were skiers, but one woman was not. She had tried cross-country skiing, without success, and even Aspen's

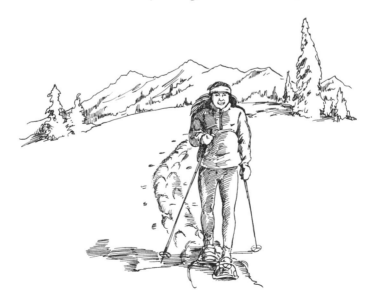

crossing an open meadow in the mountains

exemplary shopping had finally bored her. Snowshoeing proved to be her introduction to the Rocky Mountain winter world. A scenic 15-minute gondola ride to the Aspen Mountain summit was the beginning of her adventure.

On one of those perfect Western days, with sparkling sunshine, blue skies, and not a breath of wind, we snowshoed southward from the gondola terminal, leaving the realm of Alpine skiing behind. We moved single-file through the deep snow in measured steps, stopping every time Rebecca saw a large or small wonder along the way that merited an explanation, which was frequent. She talked about mountain weather systems and the formations of snow crystals, about the vegetation that grows at the 10,600-foot summit elevation, about the animals that live there and what we can infer from the tracks they leave, about the geology and the mineralogy, about the human impact of miners, loggers, and skiers on the mountainscape. She gave her talks against the gorgeous backdrop of the Aspen Highlands ski area across Castle Creek Valley and the Maroon Bells beyond. We were all captivated by Rebecca's interpretive tour, none of us more so than the non-skier in the group. She handled the snowshoes easily, even at Aspen Mountain's lofty elevation, and she was a convert. There, at the summit of one of Colorado's magnificent mountains, I witnessed the conversion of a lowlander into someone who had learned that "Winter Feels Good." She planned to return to the Nordic center and snowshoe some more and I was sure that when the foursome planned their next winter trip together, she was far less likely to suggest going on a cruise because she had discovered the beauty of winter in the high country.

Taking a tour, as this group did with the ACES program, is, for many people, the ideal introduction to snowshoeing. All sorts of outdoor clubs, social organizations from singles' to seniors' clubs, recreation centers, and adult education programs have put snowshoeing events on their winter calendars, and beginners are usually encouraged to sign up. Elderhostel offers multi-day snowshoeing programs that feature ecological programs and a gentle introduction to the sport for older adventurers with different levels of fitness. Snowshoeing is increasingly finding its way into local winter festivals in mountain towns, where downhill ski resorts and cross-country centers now offer snowshoeing. Many outdoor retail stores that sell or rent snowshoes host what are called "demo days," during which you can try equipment and get a few of those snowshoeing tips, as well as clinics, workshops, guided snowshoe walks, or in-store slide shows on the subject. Check local newspapers for listings of snowshoeing activities. For links to local hiking and outdoor groups, many of which offer guided hikes and introductions to snowshoeing programs, go to the American Hiking Society's main Web site and click on the Alliance of Hiking Organizations button (see Resources, page 132), for Web site). Even local chapters of backcountry, mountaineering, and conservation organizations such as the Appalachian Mountain Club, the Colorado Mountain Club, and the Sierra Club offer snowshoeing events, though some are more gonzo than introductory.

L. L. Bean, which started outfitting New England outdoorsmen in 1912 with the introduction of hunting footwear that quickly gained renown as "the Bean boot," organizes seasonal snowshoeing demo activities from its Freeport, Maine, flagship store. Anyone who visits on a winter weekend can sign up for a quick and efficient introduction to snowshoeing. Bean's free Walk-On Adventures program includes transportation to nearby Fogg Farm and a small-group snowshoeing immersion. I occasionally flew into Portland, Maine, when visiting my son who was going to school in New Hampshire. On a gray winter weekend, I detoured to Bean's and impulsively registered for a snowshoeing session on the farm. For me, it proved to be a nice little leg-stretcher between the airplane ride and the drive across the state line, and I was impressed by the friendly care the staff showed in giving tentative new snowshoers a thorough and informative introduction to the sport.

The biggest demo day of all is Winter Trails Day, a one-day extravaganza sponsored by SnowSports Industries America and the American Hiking Society. It takes place at about 100 locations all over the snowbelt and offers a free introduction to snowshoeing. Many manufacturers and/or retailers offer free use of demo equipment and provide snowshoeing tips and perhaps short interpretive snowshoe walks, often accompanied by a festive winter-carnival-type atmosphere. Nordic centers across the north country offer use of snowshoes, suspend trail fees, conduct guided snowshoe walks, or some combination. Most Winter Trails Day venues schedule theirs in mid-January, with Colorado's Rocky Mountain National Park traditionally putting its on a month later, in mid-February. This schedule can change, so be sure to check by logging on to the Winter Trails Day Web site (see Resources, page 132) or simply keeping your eyes open for Winter Trails Day information in your local newspaper or promotional material at nearby sporting-goods stores. When it debuted in 1997 with little fanfare, Winter Trails Day attracted more than 2,000 people to community parks, nature centers, and public lands whose recreation trails are used for snowshoeing. Now, Rocky Mountain National Park alone welcomes that many snowshoeing debutants.

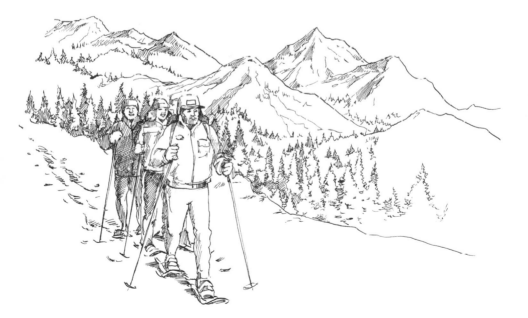

group of snowshoers on ranger-led tour

Interpretive tours are ideal for getting out into the winter environment and are part of the winter programs at many wildlife sanctuaries. A good place to start is the National Audubon Society's Web site (see Resources, page 132). Snowshoe tours have also become a staple with mountaineering/outdoors/conservation groups. Some of the best opportunities for snowshoe hikes are offered by rangers or other naturalists in snowbelt national parks. In some cases, advance reservations are required. The National Park Service's Web site (see Resources, page 132) contains links to all individual park sites. The format can change, so check with the specific park. You can also find selected programs in Appendix A.

Snowshoeing guides based at mountain resorts lead excursions on quiet trails within the boundaries of the lift-served ski area or nearby and cater to resort guests. Steamboat, Colorado, for example offers a great gourmet snowshoe hike including a fine lunch at Ragnar's Restaurant, an on-mountain restaurant of considerable local renown. You will also find some of these resort excursions in Appendix B. Naturalist guides teach about winter ecology in the mountains and show clients how to identify animal tracks in the snow. Hiking and climbing guides have found a winter niche, customizing snowshoe tours for any level of fitness or experience, from timid novices to veterans who want to learn about winter camping and mountaineering. Some offer avalanche safety courses for snowshoers with backcountry ambitions. Easy ways to find these guides are through local visitor centers, chambers of commerce, or local outdoor retail stores.

Finding Your Way

Getting lost in summer is usually not such a big deal. Daylight hours run well into the evening, it usually doesn't get horrifically cold, in most locales it probably won't snow (let alone blizzard), and there are likely to be other hikers on the trail to point you in the right direction. Winter is a whole other story. The thrill of exploring the winter wilderness becomes too thrilling if you get lost. Chapter five discusses the basic aspects of backcountry wilderness survival in case you ever do get in trouble, but remember that the overwhelming majority of snowshoers don't get seriously lost or stranded. You do leave an obvious set of tracks when snowshoeing, and unless fast-falling or blowing snow obscures them, you can usually retrace your route. Still, if you don't have a clue as to where you are going, you *could* be following someone else's tracks!

When it comes to the backcountry, especially in winter, I believe in such old adages as "Practice makes perfect" and "Old habits die hard." Practice good habits until they get old, or at least automatic. Always load your pack with the crucial basics for every outing and follow certain patterns, whether or not you are familiar with a trail and no matter what the weather. In addition to this trio of basic tips for finding your way, further information for increasing safety and enjoyment on every snowshoe hike is detailed below:

▲ Plan your hike, and tell someone where you are going and when you intend to return so they will know if you're significantly late, and be especially on the lookout if the weather has turned. (A fallback is to write down your intended route and how many are in your party, seal the paper in a plastic zip bag, and tuck it under the windshield wiper when you park your car at a trailhead.)

▲ Carry a map of the area where you plan to hike (see below) and a compass.

▲ Always hike in a group or with at least one other adult companion and perhaps a winter-worthy dog, if permitted.

Snowshoeing routes are of three basic types. On an out-and-back trail, you start at a trailhead, go to the end or as far as you wish, turn around, and return to the same trailhead. A loop route can either be one continuous trail that begins and ends at the same trailhead, or a combination of trails that eventually bring you back where you started. A shuttle trail, which stretches between two trailheads, requires two cars and two drivers.

The first "tool" for hikers, year-round, is lightweight and folds easily into pack or pocket. It is, of course, a good map. Unless you are snowshoeing along a familiar and foolproof route, say, from your vacation retreat up the country lane and back again, you need a map. When you and your companions have selected a trail (perhaps from a guidebook, ranger or information office, or on the advice of a friend), be sure to get an accurate and appropriate topographic map and read it before you start snowshoeing. The factors to consider before setting out are the total trail distance, the elevation gain, the weather and snow conditions, and the stamina and range of the slowest, weakest person in your group. On an out-and-back trail, distance is not so much of an issue, because you can turn around anytime and retrace your steps, remembering that the turn-around point is one-half of your total hiking distance. If you started walking uphill, the return will prove to be the easier half, but you might be more tired by then. On a loop trail or a shuttle hike, you are halfway home to the trailhead once you have passed the midpoint, and there's no benefit in turning back. In any event, check your map as you are going and pay particular attention at trail intersections, which might be well marked, poorly marked, not marked at all, or have signs buried in the snow.

My favorite maps for hiking, summer or winter, are the National Geographic *Trails Illustrated* series, available online or through their catalog (see Resources, page 132, for ordering information). These maps are based on United States Geological Survey topographic maps, revised and updated in coordination with the United States Forest Service, the United States Bureau of Land Management, and other agencies. Printed in color on moisture- and rip-resistant material, they are full of useful details for backcountry travel. Contour lines that show elevations, roads (both those with year-round vehicular use and unplowed roads that become part of the winter trail system), trails (the best winter trails marked with a Nordic skier icon), streams, lakes, reservoirs, wetlands and marshes, forested and tree-free areas, towns and townsites, jurisdiction boundaries for public lands, backcountry huts, and more are printed clearly. States mapped by *Trails Illustrated* that offer reliable snowshoeing include Alaska, California, Colorado, Maine, Michigan, Montana, Nevada, New Hampshire, New Mexico, Oregon, South Dakota, Utah, Vermont, Washington, Wisconsin, and Wyoming. There are also dedicated recreational maps to Yellowstone and Yosemite National Parks. Comparable maps for the most popular areas in the Canadian Rockies are issued by Gem Trek Maps (see Resources, page 132, for ordering information) with winter-specific trails shown on some of the maps.

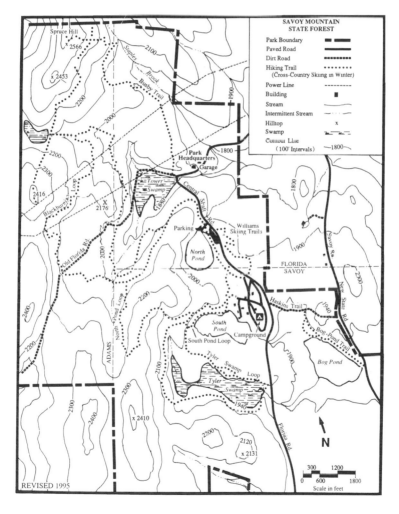

topographical contour map

Public land management agencies also issue dedicated maps, some specifically showing winter trails. These might be maps of an individual local, state, or county park or wildlife refuge, or even the route of a single specific trail. The U.S. Park Service often supplements glossy fold-out maps, available at the visitor center and entrance station of every land parcel under its management with useful specific winter trail maps. The Forest Service also prints up free winter-specific information sheets on individual trails. Each handout includes such information as a route map, direction to the trailhead, length, elevation gain, perhaps a trail profile, verbal description, degree of challenge, cautions (stream crossings, avalanche potential, and possible weather hazards), and other helpful data. This material may also be available on the Forest Service Web site. This is helpful because most of the agency's offices are closed on weekends and holidays, which is when most people go out snowshoeing. Nordic centers provide trail maps of their own systems. Routes are usually well signed as well, providing an excellent opportunity to practice navigation skills by relating signs to maps. Many guidebooks also have specific route maps for each trail described. Make a photocopy of the relevant page, or several, so that each person in your party has one.

Another useful backcountry tool is a compass, but be sure you know how to use it. When the needle swings to "north," it is pointing toward the magnetic pole. To know which way is true north, you need to adjust it to the geographic pole, on which topo maps are based. *Trails Illustrated* and similar maps feature a clock-like graphic that shows how many degrees the compass needs to be adjusted for the longitude covered on that map. Lay your compass on top of the graphic, and rotate the bezel to match. (Taking a compass-reading workshop, perhaps at an adult-education center or outdoor shop, is helpful, and practicing these skills, summer or winter, is a good idea.) Especially when snow obscures landmarks along the route, your compass and map will give you an idea of where you might be on a trail that twists and turns. In mountainous areas, an altimeter is a useful accessory, too. Matching the altimeter reading with the contour lines on your map can help you figure out your location, but remember that it must be reset every day to match the elevation at the trailhead and also that changes in barometric pressure during your hike can throw off the accurate elevation reading.

We are living in the age of the backcountry techno-geek. People tote Global Positioning System (GPS) units and cell phones into the backcountry, expecting them to answer all their questions and solve all their problems. But just as a telephone or electric line can go down or a computer can crash, these instruments have their limitations, especially in mountainous areas or in deep valleys and canyons, where satellite contact can be difficult or impossible. Batteries can weaken or die. Furthermore, while a GPS can pinpoint your location, it can't lead you from where you are to where you want to go as reliably or simply as a map can. The bottom line, in my view, is that if you love gadgets, take them along and get accustomed to using them, but always take the compact, lightweight, reliable map and compass.

Trail Etiquette

Much the way summer roads are used by motor vehicles, cyclists, runners, and walkers, the reality of winter recreation is that the great majority of routes are multi-use, so snowshoers need to be mindful of sharing the "road" with skiers and perhaps snowmobilers. No matter who is on the trail, the basic advice for snowshoers is: Follow the posted rules. This is equally true at Nordic centers, Alpine ski areas, and other commercial venues. On public lands, common courtesy and safety dictate obeying certain guidelines, for in the winter world, snowshoers are at the bottom of the food chain. Nordic skiers move faster than snowshoers on the downhills — and snowmobiles are faster still. Self-preservation for snowshoers means being aware of and considerate of other users and stepping out of the way when necessary.

The Forest Service and other public lands administrators have a pretty loose policy on where nonmotorized users are legally permitted to go and what they are legally permitted to do. For ease of route-finding and safety, most new snowshoers tend to stick to established and marked routes, but in most cases, it isn't mandatory. You are permitted to strike out on your own, bushwhacking or climbing straight up to high ridges if you care to. On snowshoes, you have the ability and freedom to do so. In spring, summer, and fall, erosion-prone "social trails" can be created by many boots walking on the same strip of often-fragile soil, but this is not a problem in winter, when snow insulates every plantlet from snowshoers' footfalls. Public roads, however, and sometimes even trails connecting the trailhead to a big forest parcel can be rights-of-way flanked by private land. If a sign says, "Private Property — No Trespassing," respect the private property, obey the sign, and don't trespass, even if the land feels wild and uninhabited.

Snowshoers and Nordic skiers often share the same trails but not the same activity. This can cause conflicts. The biggest single issue that Nordic skiers have with snowshoers is that the latter sometimes tramp down the tracks that the former have etched into the snow. In the backcountry, the first skier to break trail sets a pair of parallel tracks in new snow, often at great effort, especially on the uphill, expecting the reward of a fast, smooth downhill run on the return. They have every right to get upset when unthinking snowshoers walk on their tracks, chopping them up and making for a less pleasurable downhill run. If skiers have gone first, snowshoe next to, rather than on, the ski tracks. If you are first, snowshoe along one side of the trail, not right down the middle, so that skiers have room to lay down tracks too. Once a number of snowshoers and skiers have used a particular trail, this is less of an issue because snowshoes, skis, poles, and skiers will have tramped the snow down, eradicating any ski tracks.

Sharing roads with snowmobilers is a whole different situation. Most snowshoers don't relish hiking along well-used snowmobile routes because the snowmachines' noise and exhaust are simply not pleasant. On relatively quiet weekdays, routes from more remote trailheads, or other places less popular with snowmobilers, this is less of an issue. Though we all have our degree of tolerance, I personally don't have a problem being occasionally passed by snowmobiles. I step aside and wave. They give me and other snowshoers a decent berth and wave back. I find that their passing packs down the snow and makes easier going on snowshoes, but not all my snowshoeing companions are as snow-mobile-tolerant as I am. In fact, some absolutely refuse to consider a trail that also is used for mechanized recreation.

Cross-country skiing and snowshoeing are more compatible. At established cross-country centers, a set of parallel, ski-width "classical tracks" is mechanically etched into the snow for skiers to follow and snowshoers to stay off. Some cross-country centers ask snowshoers to stay on the "skating lanes," which are wide, trackless trails, and other ski areas provide designated snowshoeing trails. Still others prohibit

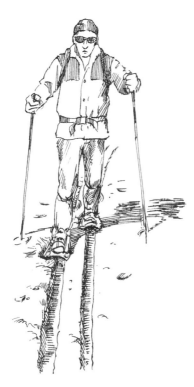

snowshoer stepping on
cross-country ski tracks (incorrect)

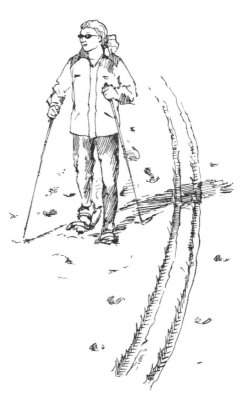

snowshoer walking beside
ski tracks (correct)

snowshoeing entirely to prevent conflict. Some Nordic centers request that snowshoers stick to only dedicated snowshoe trails, stay on the skating lanes of groomed cross-country trails, or snowshoe beside the groomed portion of the trails. Most cross-country trails are laid out as one-way, and many can be assembled into loops. Be sure to travel in the designated direction, and don't move against the traffic. If you are snowshoeing on skating lanes, stay near the outside edge of the groomed section and be mindful of fast-moving skate-skiers coming up behind you. Customarily, they yell "track" when gaining on you, but you might not hear them or, if you are in mid-lane, you might not hear them quickly enough to move out of the way.

Some Alpine ski areas permit snowshoeing within the boundaries, some even conduct snowshoeing tours there, and a few permit snowshoers to ride one or more lifts to access on-mountain routes. Ski areas that permit snowshoeing understandably regulate where, and sometimes when, snowshoers may go. Some resorts have snowshoe trails interwoven among their downhill trails, others permit snowshoeing on easier, green-circle routes that are often snow-covered roads that in summer provide vehicular access. Some permit snowshoeing only early in the morning, before the lifts start operating. Again, whatever the rules are, follow them.

Children, Seniors, and Canine Companions

Snowshoeing is a wonderful family activity, one that you can start before children are actually capable of taking a step of their own. In fact, you moms-to-be can snowshoe even before your baby is born. The stable platform that snowshoes provide is a fine way for pregnant women to get some fresh air and exercise in winter. Once the baby has arrived, snowshoeing offers an excellent winter activity for new parents. On mild, wind-free days, outdoorsy parents bundle up their babies, slather sunscreen on their little faces, tuck them into a Snuggly (if they're small) or a baby backpack (if they're bigger) and head off for a modest

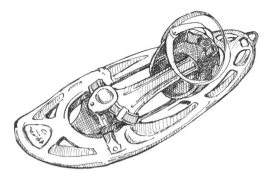

one-piece all-plastic snowshoe

snowshoe walk. The gentle soft-step motion of parental snowshoeing lulls many a baby to sleep and, if you keep your hike fairly short, you should be back at the trailhead before the baby is hungry.

Preschoolers love to play in the snow, so low-level, age-appropriate snowshoeing activities are a natural. Snowshoe manufacturers have complied by making small models designed for lightweight youngsters. What is unnatural is expecting them to go on a snowshoe *hike.* Far better to plan a short walk with plenty of time to play in the snow, make snow angels, build a snowman, or go sledding. In fact, savvy parents take a sled along not just for sliding down a small hill somewhere along the way, but for towing a tired child back to the trailhead. In addition to snowshoes, snow-wear, and snacks, remember to take extra mittens and hats because the ones they started out with are sure to get wet or less likely to get lost. Snowed-in campgrounds and roadside picnic areas are great venues for families with small children. Even if the main site is unplowed, highway crews usually plow a pullout for parking. The ground is relatively flat, and there are wide, safe spaces between campsites and picnic tables. Some have raised grills that can be dusted (or shoveled) off, so on nice days, even consider bringing some charcoal and fire-starter and grilling some food as part of the treat.

School-age children can begin really snowshoeing. Start with a moderate hike of no more than a mile and be ready to stop, play, and explore. Some youngsters do best in a WABP (with anyone but parents) situation. The minimum age for guided snowshoe hikes in many venues is eight, and often even the kid who won't cooperate with or listen to parents will hang on every word and follow every step of a guide or park ranger in a spiffy uniform.

Compared with even the smallest adult models, child-size snowshoes look really tiny and sometimes downright flimsy. The size is fine, because lightweight children don't need a large snowshoe for flotation. Rugged plastic snowshoes are also fine for children playing in the snow and walking short distances. The smallest snowshoes are colorful plastic ones shaped into ovals that mimic old snowshoe webbing or animal paws. There are no metal crampons to cause injury when youngsters are rolling around in the snow. Older children use snowshoes that are smaller, lighter versions of adult shoes. In selecting kids' snowshoes, the priority should be finding easy-to-buckle (and -unbuckle) bindings (though your little one might be more interested in the color of the plastic or the shape of the decking). Adjust the bindings to your child's boot at home so that you aren't trying to figure out which way the strap fits into the buckle when you're ready to go out on the trail. If possible, do a practice round. It's better, but not mandatory for there to be snow on the ground. Go outside, fit the bindings to the boots, and let your child walk around in the yard to get the feel of the gear.

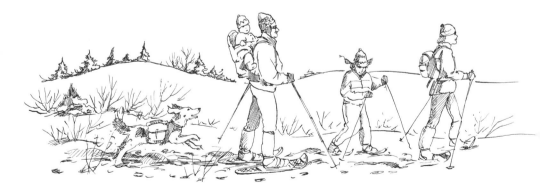

snowshoeing as a family activity

Many special snowshoeing events include something for children — perhaps a family fun race, nature adventure, or other activity that are broad in their appeal. For example, the Black Bear Lodge on Little St. Germain Lake, Wisconsin, produces the annual Snow Blaze, a family-oriented event with snowshoe treks, guided hikes, and a roaring campfire with hot dogs, brats, and marshmallows cooking away for hungry youngsters and their parents. Smiling Hill Farm, a 500-acre dairy farm in Westbrook, Maine, offers the usual snowshoeing trails, snack bar, and such, but also sleigh rides and animal exhibits. Parents and children may enjoy a family snowshoe weekend at Treehaven, a field station between Rhinelander and Tomahawk, Wisconsin. Among the programs offered by the University of Wisconsin, Stevens Point, is a snowshoeing opportunity for children aged 5 to 10 and their parents to join an experienced adventure education instructor for a weekend of winter snowshoe hiking on UWSP's 1,400 acres of northern forest. The Hills Ranch at 108 Mile, British Columbia, has 20 family-style chalets, 26 lodge rooms, a phenomenal cross-country system, a 1,000-acre "snowshoe park," and other activities that range from tubing to snowmobiling to sliding on a lighted on-site ski hill.

Likewise, seniors enjoy ample opportunities to snowshoe. This healthy, low-impact, do-it-at-your-own-pace activity is ideal for preventing or rolling back an assortment of ailments. It also lends itself to the small-group recreation that is so popular with active seniors. In Colorado, for instance, Durango-based Seniors Outdoors weaves snowshoeing outings into its full program of summer hiking, biking, and whitewater rafting and winter Nordic and Alpine skiing. The senior program at the East Boulder Recreation Center runs a weekly bus to Eldora Mountain Resort, where participants have a choice of downhill or cross-country skiing or, increasingly, snowshoeing. Other programs in other snowbelt communities also put snowshoeing on their calendars, and with health-conscious, leading-edge baby boomers moving solidly into the seniors category, snowshoeing's popularity will only increase. Unlike children, whose special needs tend to be along the lines of preventing boredom, about the only precautions that seniors need to take is to keep warm (some might get cold faster than younger adults) and to pace themselves if their energy reserves aren't what they once were.

Several years ago, while researching a Colorado snowshoeing guidebook, one of my destinations was Crested Butte. In this small town, somebody told somebody who told somebody that I was coming, and by the time I arrived, I was invited to join a group of active retirees who had a standing weekly date to hike, which in winter meant on snowshoes. On a gray deep-winter day, with a steady breeze blowing snow clouds into the valley, we formed up at the Crested Butte Nordic Center and quickly set off on the Green Lake Trail. The leader set a good pace, and after a while we veered off into woods to a sheltered clearing. We stopped in a quiet spot with snow falling softly on our shoulders. The only sound was the click of plastic buckles releasing and packs sliding off shoulders. My new friends stood their packs upright in a circle in the snow — a small Stonehenge of colored Cordura. The next sound was pack zippers being opened, and the next sight was of delicious treasures emerging. One woman bakes bread. Another cookies. Someone is in charge of *charcuterie* (sausage) and cheese. Someone else always brings olives and others condiments. One man is in charge of wine. Someone brings paper and plastic and a trash bag for the leavings. We toasted and tasted, and I was made to feel as welcome as if I had been part of the group forever.

For many outdoors lovers, no snowshoeing buddy surpasses a canine companion. If you take your dog hiking in summer, you already know this. "I've never met a dog who doesn't love frolicking in the snow," said Cindy Hirschfeld, who with her golden retriever, Clover, has hiked thousands of miles to research her book, *Canine Colorado.* "Clover loves to porpoise under deep snow drifts. She rolls on her back and makes doggie snow angels. She buries her head in the snow and tunnels. Dog owners get as much joy from watching their dogs romp in the snow as from any other part of a winter hike."

When you plan your excursion, be sure that dogs are permitted on the route you choose. They are welcome on most Forest Service and Bureau of Land Management lands, including wilderness areas but excluding some national recreation areas. Many, but not all, national parks and preserves also prohibit dogs, but where they are allowed, they must be leashed. State parks and provincial parks have their own regulations. Leash laws elsewhere vary — and they may vary by county. Check whether dogs may be under voice command or must be leashed. Regardless of how a dog is controlled, be sure to pick up any waste the dog deposits on the trail. Even if it's snowing and you think the dog's leavings will soon be covered, imagine how you would feel stepping in it. Off-trail and out-of-sight piles will generally decompose naturally before they gross anyone else out.

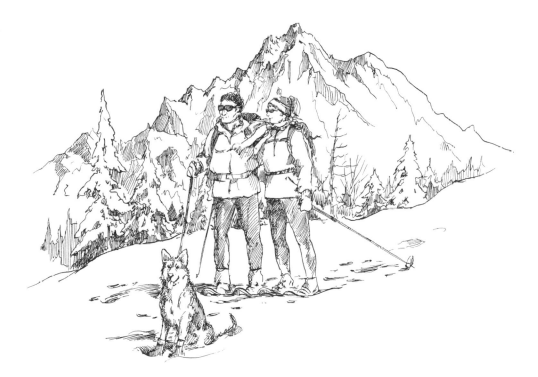

snowshoeing in the backcountry

Big, thick-coated dogs that love snow and cold are wonderful snow-shoeing buddies. Short-haired breeds or dogs with small, dainty paws aren't designed for winter hikes and dogs with webbed feet need special considerations when heading out in the snow, but long-haired dogs bred to work in cold weather are fabulous on the trail. Huskies and malamutes, of course, are naturals in the winter environment. Labs, retrievers, and German shepherds are large and sturdy enough for winter hikes. One caution: Ice balls tend to build up in their paws. Ice can cut a dog's feet and even some hard, abrasive snow can cause tiny fissures in pads. Some people spray Pam or other vegetable anti-stick cooking spray directly on their paws. Pet stores and dog boutiques carry several brands of special booties, and some dog-owners swear by a product called Musher's Secret Wax. This soft, fast-drying, wax-based cream is applied to the dog's pads, between its toes and pads, and between its toes to form a semi-permeable shield that sheds snow, protects paws, and acts like an invisible boot.

In addition to being energetic and enthusiastic companions, dogs provide a level of loyalty and backcountry security that is hard to beat. Your dog will stay with you through thick and thin (which might mean thick snowfall or thin air) and is a real comfort if the going gets tough. Winter-savvy dogs will grab a mouthful of snow when they are thirsty, a practice not recommended for their humans. Be sure to bring enough food for your dog (dry treats will do), and mind the rules about where dogs are permitted and whether they must be leashed. Again, as a courtesy to those who follow, remove any dog waste from the trail. And just as you courteously avoid snowshoeing over cross-country tracks, try to keep your dog off them, too.

five

Kicking It Up

*Racing, backcountry exploring, and other
snowshoe adventures*

All that many snowshoers ever want from the sport is a gentle walk in the woods or a pleasant nature hike, but for others, that is just the beginning. They want to go faster or farther or embark on more adventurous snowshoe excursions. Earlier, I observed that whatever you can do in the summer on bare ground is possible on snowshoes when there's snow. Runners run on snowshoes, and backpackers backpack on snowshoes. (Confession time. I don't run, and I don't winter camp, so unlike those that have preceded it, this chapter does not reflect my personal experiences.) Thousands of snowshoers run, race, and spend winter nights under rip-stop nylon or in a snow cave. I also know that snowshoeing on any level is a way to become stronger and healthier. So if getting or staying in shape is one of your goals, read on.

About the Nighthawk Racing Series at Eldora Mountain Resort in Nederland, Colorado, Mike Sandrock, running columnist for the *Boulder Daily Camera,* wrote, "Don't expect the fastest road runners to be coming in first . . . Running on snowshoes requires much more energy than running on dry roads." Does it ever! The rule of thumb is that snowshoeing burns about 25 percent more calories than dry land locomotion at a comparable speed and type of terrain. According to two studies, walking just 2.4 miles per hour on snowshoes on a flat, packed trail burns 420 calories. Add powder snow, and a woman snowshoeing at 3.3 miles per hour on a flat trail will typically burn 744 calories; a man, 984. Put on a pack or a toddler in a backpack or snowshoe on hilly terrain, and the calorie expenditure increases. It gets even better for runners. Running 5.2 miles per hour on a flat trail uses an average of 570 calories per hour, and a racing speed of 7.5 miles per hour burns 890 calories.

Aggressive snowshoeing at altitude, in deep snow, or with speed provides such an effective aerobic workout that *The Berkeley Wellness Letter* pegged it as "nearly as good a cardiovascular workout as stairclimbing." In addition to being heart-healthy, snowshoeing is a great muscle toner that has additional cross-training benefits for endurance sportsters: Aggressive snowshoeing helps build the quads, the hamstrings, and the calf muscles. Climbing hills on snowshoes works the hip flexors and extensors, which are used for cycling. Adding poles increases the calorie burn and helps work the shoulders, chest, and triceps. Since energy expenditure translates to greater fitness, and walking or hiking on snowshoes requires more energy than walking or hiking on dry ground, it's clear that even in its mellowest form, snowshoeing is great exercise, and at a high level, it is unsurpassed for fitness.

Run, Snowshoer, Run

The continuum from snowshoeing and running and eventually to racing is direct. Mountain runner and Redfeather founder Bill Perkins, who was instrumental in refining today's aluminum-frame snowshoes, is widely acknowledged as the forefather of today's snowshoe running and racing craze. When lightweight snowshoes became the norm, running really took off. When people run, some inevitably race, hence the abundance of organized competitions and the possibility that snowshoe racing will eventually become a winter Olympic sport.

Snowshoe running in the modern era started as and remains a natural winter cross-training activity for serious road and mountain runners and multi-sport endurance athletes. Thanks to the cushioning nature of the snow, it is low-impact, yet it helps maintain or enhance aerobic capacity and keep the muscles toned. Distance runners, who are accustomed to the pounding they take on asphalt, quickly appreciate the forgiveness of snow under their feet and the freedom of flying downhill by adding a little glissade to every step. There are a few technique tweaks: When snowshoeing, runners must remember to pick their feet up higher than they would on dry land, and they might have to adjust their foot strike to get the most traction from the claws. Experts recommend that runners transitioning to snowshoes start on packed trails rather than in loose snow. Runners usually adjust easily to snowshoeing on packed trails, though they are often surprised that their speed diminishes. "If you're a runner or triathlete, snowshoe running is a great way to stay race-fit during the winter months. While your running gait might seem awkward at first, you'll get enormous cardiovascular benefits from it. And when you're sweltering in the hot mid-July sun, you can recall your snowshoe running to help keep you cool," says Brian Metzler, a serious endurance athlete and editor of *Adventure Sports* magazine.

Athletes recovering from injury also benefit from snowshoeing, not just to rebuild endurance and strength but also because soft snow is kind to bones and joints, even as it builds muscles and endurance. Snowshoes designed for running are small (about 8 by 25 inches) and lightweight (generally under 3 pounds and sometimes closer to 2 pounds). They feature reliable traction devices, often asymmetrical frame shapes, and bindings that fit over running or cross-training footwear. For packed snow, the decking may be of a more open design to reduce weight. For powder, full decking fills more area within the frame for greater

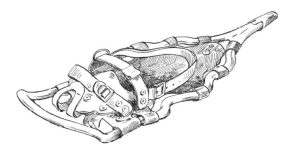

racing snowshoe

flotation. Trail runners tend to prefer fixed toe-cord bindings, because when they pick up their feet, their snowshoes do not drag on the snow, while rotating toe cords are often favored for off-trail running because they quickly shed snow that would add weight.

Some snowshoes for running come with insulated bindings, but because serious racers often attach running shoes directly to the snowshoes and eliminate the binding altogether, they've also devised several tricks for keeping their feet warm and dry. One method is to pull cycling booties over running shoes. Another is to wear neoprene socks under or neoprene spats over regular shoes. Still another is to wear two pairs of socks with plastic bags between them, but since the plastic traps moisture, this is not a good tactic for people whose feet perspire. Runners who use the two-socks-plus-plastic method buy larger running shoes to accommodate the extra bulk. Danelle Ballangee, a Colorado-based world-class multi-sport competitor, snowshoe racer, and personal trainer (see page vii), counsels, "If you start to feel cold, take care of it before it gets too bad."

When people start running, it seems inevitable that some begin running against each other, and thus snowshoe racing was born — or reborn. The connection between Quebec and snowshoe racing remains undiminished (see chapter one for more information). In 2004, Saint-Laurent Borough hosted the 96th International Snowshoe Championship in Parc Marcel-Laurin, attracting 150 competitors from Canada and the United States. Elsewhere, interest in snowshoe racing that had disappeared over the years has been rekindled with the boom in jogging, running, and endurance sports. In chicken-and-egg fashion, Bill Perkins developed the first made-for-running aluminum-frame snowshoe for his own running and racing, and the rise of the Redfeather company that he founded made it easier for more participants to do their running on appropriately designed snowshoes. Regional differences in snowshoe-racing styles have emerged. In the East, most snowshoe races take place on packed-snow tracks. Midwestern races are often run on packed snow too, but often include longer distances. In the West, races through untracked snow are popular, though of course, later racers don't have to break trail but benefit from the snow packed down by the swifter snowshoers who preceded them.

Even snowshoe manufacturers, enjoying the sport's booming popularity, sponsor races all over the continent. Names like Atlas, Dion, Redfeather, and Tubbs are all now associated with competitions. The North American snowshoe-racing calendar is full of races over various distances including 1-kilometer fun runs, family runs, and kids' races; the widely popular 5K and 10K events; sprints and relays; and demanding endurance races over great distances in unpacked snow. Frequently, there are snowshoeing components to multi-sport winter events. Snowshoeing lends itself to some really daunting endurance events, which are generally held in wild and in remote stretches of country. A couple of famous competitions have come and gone. Alaska's Iditashoe Snowshoe Race and the Cold Foot Classic, both 100-milers, are no longer held. But the Yukon Arctic Ultra, a multi-sport race with snowshoeing as an option for all or part of the course, takes place each February departing from and returning to Whitehorse,

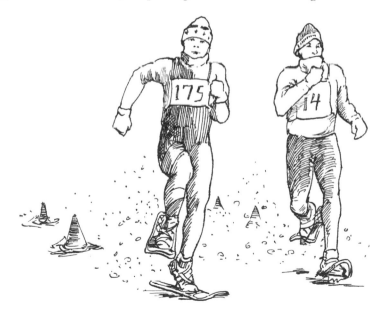

snowshoers racing

Yukon Territory. Competition distances are 100 and 300 miles. This race gives new meaning to the phrase "brutal challenge." Andrew Barnett, winner of the 300K footrace division in 2004, crossed the finish line in 6 days, 2 hours — 24 hours faster than the 2003 winner and 14 hours ahead of his two runners-up, who finished together.

The Yukon Arctic Ultra is in a class by itself, but other endurance races are difficult because of altitude and elevation gain. Such events include the Mt. Elbert Challenge up and down Colorado's highest peak (14,433 feet), with 6,000 feet of elevation change and a total distance of about 15 miles. Snowshoers now dominate America's Uphill, a grueling 3,267-foot ascent of Aspen Mountain, Colorado. The course record is under 49 minutes, which is all the more remarkable when you consider that the gondola climbs the same distance in 15 minutes.

Elite competitors seem built for speed, endurance, and mental toughness, and some snowshoeing legends appear unbeatable for years at a time. Shawn Lyons (a bearded musician, adjunct professor at the University of Alaska at Anchorage, and newspaper columnist) was a nine-time winner of the Iditashoe and three-time winner of the 100-mile Cold Foot Classic, which once took place on Halloween above the Arctic Circle. Tom Sobal (a bearded Colorado snowshoe racer, snowshoeing coach and trainer, snowshoeing writer, and race organizer) has won something on the order of 130 snowshoe races ranging from 1 to 100 miles. He is a five-time world snowshoeing champion, longtime holder of the world's best marathon time on snowshoes (3:06:17), and in the "off-season" is a trail runner whose accomplishments include three-time triple crown champion in pack burro racing with his burro, Bullwinkle. Danelle Ballangee, a Colorado-based adventure racer, trainer, and race organizer (no beard) is a formidable adventure racer and competitor in such events as the storied Ironman Triathlon. In addition to dozens of dry-land victories, she was named 1997 Duathlete of the Year and 2002 Adventure Racer of the Year. She was the 2002 National Snowshoe Champion, was undefeated in 50 consecutive snowshoe races between January 4, 1997, and January 20, 2001, and has won over one hundred snowshoe races at various distances.

Ballangee keeps in over-the-top shape by running uphill as much as possible, which she believes is the best hamstring-strengthener there is. To maximize her uphill without "wasting" time while going downhill, she has been known to sled down. If that appeals to you, but you don't want to tow a sled uphill, think about adding an Airboard to your snowshoe training gear. This inflatable sled, designed in Europe, weighs just six pounds and fits in a backpack. The downhill zoom is like riding on an air cushion, which is a lot of hoot-and-holler fun. Airboard is for open-slope use, not for wooded areas, because you ride lying prone and head-first. You may even want to don a helmet . . . just in case.

The United States Snowshoe Association, founded in 1977, is the governing body for snowshoe racing in the United States. It took 24 years after its establishment for the first National Snowshoe Championships to be held. In the interim, the USSSA established rules and standards that range from physical (how the start and finish are handled, track layout, and more) and administrative (setting responsibilities for the race coordinator and other officials), to organizational (standardizing age and gender classifications in races). It has also decided on minimum standard sizes for snowshoes used in sanctioned races (now 12 square inches, replacing the previous standard of a minimum snowshoe size of 25 by 8 inches).

The snowshoe-racing community continues to grow. The United States Snowshoe Association (see the "Organizations" list in Resources, page 132) is the best clearing house for information on races. Not only has it adopted official rules for snowshoe racing in coordination with the International Amateur Snowshoe Racing Federation, but it also maintains an event calendar, tracks race results, fields a national snowshoe racing team and in other ways tries to forge ties among American snowshoe racers. But serious racing isn't all the sport offers. Snowshoe competitions often have informal fun races for families and other casual recreationists as well as serious competitors. You will find a representative list in Appendix C, page 123.

Annual stand-alone races abound, with a number of race series leading toward championship events on various levels. Several state racing league series now serve as qualifiers for the United States National Snowshoe Championships. In 2003, the five-member National Snowshoe Team made its first overseas trip to compete in the 30th anniversary of La Ciaspolada Snowshoe Race. This 7-kilometer race in the Valle de Non near Fondo, Italy, attracts roughly 6,000 racers. World Cup-style snowshoe racing also came to the United States in 2003. Snowshoeing has been part of the Special Olympics World Winter Games since 2001.

Perhaps the most intriguing races are those leading to the biennial Arctic Winter Games (see Resources, page 132). Teams of young snowshoers to age 20 from Alaska, Yukon, Northwest Territories, Nunavit, Greenland, and other remote places in the Far North compete on strictly traditional equipment (wood and *babiche* snowshoes, and mukluks instead of high-tech boots) at distances from 100 meters to 10 kilometers. To prepare for this competition, bush villagers train and compete among themselves on this classic gear. To see youthful snowshoers competing on the timeless equipment of their ancestors in the land of the midnight sun defines the true, pure meaning of sport.

When people begin racing, those who start thinking about racing faster and more efficiently begin looking to the sport's gurus for guidance. Many of the top snowshoe racers and trainers now offer workshops, clinics, and private one-on-one coaching on such topics as conditioning, race training, and racing technique. These classes are heavily promoted locally through running clubs, fitness centers, and outdoor stores.

Staying Out for the Night

Some years ago, I read a fascinating article in the late *Snowshoer* magazine about Ken Kutac's snowshoeing adventures in the Rockies, the High Sierras, and the Cascades. Kutac was then in his late 50s, and the article described his decades-long passion for getting out and staying out. Kutac recalled winter trekking and snow camping when snowshoes were five or six feet long. They made him strong, and they made him appreciate the smaller aluminum-frame models when they came along. Not one to jump on every innovation, Kutac preferred Inuit-style mukluks to factory-made boots, and he slept in what he called "snow tents" rather than under nylon. I never met Ken Kutac, and I have no idea whether he is still out there, camping in his snow tents. I have no desire to emulate him, but the article made me think of others who love the winter outdoors, by *night* as well as by day.

For those who love to run and love to race, going faster and harder is a goal. For others, backpacking in the winter world holds great appeal because their goal is to penetrate deeper into the backcountry. It also requires careful preparation and precautions. But meeting the challenges — surviving the trek, camping in the snow, and emerging from a toasty sleeping bag and tent in the morning — is immeasurably satisfying.

If these challenges sound enticing to you, winter camping may be an unsurpassed way to immerse yourself in the snowy environment.

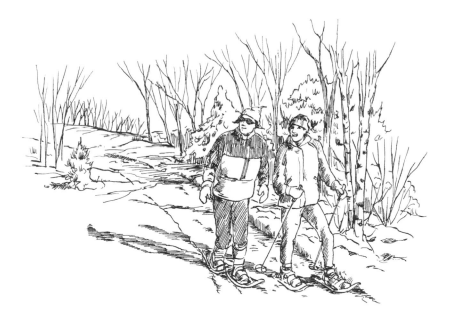

groomed, packed snowshoe trail in eastern forest

Probably the first qualification for winter camping is that you are comfortable backpacking and camping in summer. Then, it's a good idea to intentionally take some snowshoe day-hikes in adverse conditions such as extreme cold, falling snow (not a full-blown blizzard, but a snowstorm that changes visibility), and wind. Reading up on specifics of winter camping is useful, as is taking a class on winter survival and the basics of winter camping that covers winter tents, how to build a snow cave, Arctic-weight sleeping bags and insulated sleeping pads, food, hydration, waste disposal, and winter navigation. (Such classes are usually given by outdoor sports stores and by outdoor/environmental/hiking organizations.) That should get you started. For backpacking, larger-than-normal snowshoes will be needed to accommodate the extra weight of your gear, along with sturdy poles. A strong, lightweight shovel and an ice axe round out your special winter-camping gear needs. If you plan to camp off the beaten track in avalanche country (which includes anywhere in the West), it is wise to take an avalanche-awareness course. Finally, you'll probably want to try your first winter outings with an experienced friend or an organized overnight group hike led by a qualified leader or certified guide.

Navigation is, of course, more challenging in winter when new or blowing snow can fill in tracks quickly and the flat white light can be disorienting. Carrying a heavy pack through new snow is tiring, and fatigue can compound confusion over compass directions or identifying your intended route. Familiarity with map and compass reading (and if you are going high-tech, GPS use) will help. Do remember that tall trees or deep valleys can block satellite signals that GPS units rely on and batteries can die, so always carry a compass and pertinent maps.

As you hone your navigation skills, you might consider the sport of orienteering, in which participants use a compass and a detailed map to find specific, pre-selected points on the landscape. It can be a simple, low-key recreational activity or a surprisingly competitive sport. Geocaching is a high-tech version of orienteering with a hide-and-seek component. Participants use GPS units to locate caches of various

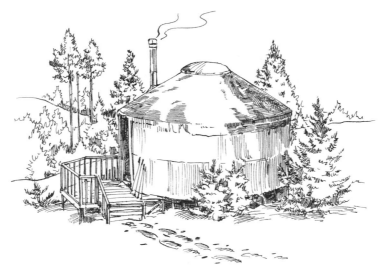

yurt warming hut

treasures, as hidden objects are called. "Hardcore geocachers are put off by very little," says Erik Sherman, author of *Geocaching: Hike and Seek with Your GPS*. "Tromping through thigh-high snow can make the activity far harder. Strapping on a pair of snowshoes is a practical answer, besides giving someone a chance to combine the challenge of seeking caches with the obvious fun of snowshoeing."

All the cautions laid out for new snowshoers in chapter three are magnified when venturing into the deep backcountry, and even more so for an overnight excursion. The detailed requirements of winter camping are beyond the scope of this book, but it is important to bear in mind that taking too casual an approach to winter conditions can, in the backcountry, have terrible consequences. A balmy daytime temperature can plummet when the sun goes down. The wind can pick up and start blowing and drifting snow. Snow can fall quickly and deeply, obscuring landmarks. Blowing snow and winter fog can cause a whiteout, in which it is difficult to discern the difference between earth and sky. If you're not amply prepared for the extremes of winter weather, you can get into a heap of trouble.

For some adventurers, snowshoeing is but one of many winter skills that they possess. Mountaineers, for instance, snowshoe on the approach for winter peak ascents — and sometimes on the mountain itself. Ellen Miller, a Colorado climber who summited Mount Everest twice in a single year via different routes and has taken part in three Mount McKinley expeditions, says that about half of the people on McKinley now use snowshoes instead of skis. This amazed me at first, because I know that climbers must make several trips to ferry their gear from the airplane landing area to the first camp. Being able to ski back down to the landing area seemed a lot easier than walking both ways. "A lot of people doing McKinley can't ski well enough with heavy packs, so they use snowshoes," she told me.

In one respect, though, winter camping is actually easier than summer camping: There are far fewer visitors in national parks and other public lands, which means you can enjoy surprising solitude much closer to a road or trailhead than in summer. While snowshoeing up Fall River Road in Rocky Mountain National Park beyond the winter closure, I encountered two Grizzly Adams-looking men on their way down, heavy backpacks on their backs and hard-to-read expressions on their faces. I envisioned their raw adventure with a precarious campsite in the alpine zone six or seven miles up the road. When I asked where they had camped, they said they'd camped just a mile away and just off the road, an area passed by hundreds of cars a day in summer. In winter, however, even Rocky Mountain National Park provides the feeling of wilderness close to "civilization."

And for those not quite prepared for full-blown winter camping, there's a kind of middle ground between a snowshoeing day trip and backpack roughing it. Consider a snowshoe trip to a backcountry hut or yurt that combines the beauty and isolation of camping with the comfort and safety of a winterized, heated shelter, perhaps one with running water, a cookstove, and some kind of toilet facility. Hut systems like Colorado's Tenth Mountain Division, Alfred Braun, and San Juan Hut Systems can be found in many state and provincial parks. However far you want to go with snowshoeing, it is the best key to appreciating the outdoors during the underappreciated winter season.

appendix A

PUBLIC LANDS

Your tax money supports local, county, state, and national parks, so you might as well use them year-round. In many parks, summer hiking trails become snowshoeing trails in winter. In other places, particularly in the far north or at very high elevations, snowshoeing routes follow frozen, snow covered streams or traverse lakes or reservoirs. Unplowed county or local roads or roads in wildlife and nature preserves look and feel remote and ethereal in winter. Other tracts administered by fish and game agencies or other conservation agencies also provide snowshoers with places to explore. And remember that in large cities and resort towns alike, snowshoeing is possible in urban and town parks and on snow-covered recreation trails.

The most extensive network of marked winter trails in the United States is found on **United States Forest Service**-administered land. There, routes marked with orange diamonds are available for both motorized (that is, snowmobiles) and nonmotorized (that is, snowshoers and Nordic skiers) uses. Routes marked with blue diamonds, including those that approach designated wilderness areas, are for nonmotorized use only. Except in only a handful of heavily traveled fee-demonstration areas, use of these forest roads is free. For specific trail information, visit the Forest Service Web site (see Resources, page 132).

National parks in the snowbelt also offer abundant snowshoeing opportunities, often including regularly scheduled ranger-guided snowshoe hikes. These are either free or are conducted with the request of a modest donation. Some park service concessionaires also offer guided tours. Contact the park before you go because reservations might be required and children younger than a certain age might not be permitted. The **United States National Park Service's** Web site (see Resources, page 132) has links to individual parks. Among the snowshoe tours available in national parks are as follows:

Crater Lake National Park, Oregon. With average annual snowfall of 533 inches, snowshoes are essential for exploring this park in winter. Ranger-led interpretive walks are presented in the Rim Village area early afternoon every Saturday and Sunday from Thanksgiving weekend through late March. Snowshoes included. Phone 541-594-3100.

Craters of the Moon National Monument and Preserve, Idaho. Ecology programs, given on midwinter Saturdays, combine 45- to 60-minute classroom sessions with two to three hours on the snow. Snowshoes available. Phone 208-527-3257.

Glacier National Park, Montana. Private outfitters offering guided snowshoe tours into the park in the winter-accessible southern portion are Glacier Park Ski Tours and Izaak Walton Inn. Phone 406-888-7800.

Grand Teton National Park, Wyoming. Ranger-led interpretive tours depart from the Moose Visitor Center. Snowshoes included. Phone 307-734-3399.

Lassen Volcanic National Park, California. Two-hour ranger-led interpretive hikes are given on Saturdays from Lassen Chalet. Snowshoes available. Phone 530-595-4444, Ext. 1.

Mount Rainier National Park, Washington. Park rangers conduct two-hour naturalist tours on winter weekends and daily during the holidays. Sign up at the Jackson Visitor Center at Paradise. Snowshoes available. Phone 360-569-2211, extension 3314. Rainier Ski Touring, a commercial guiding service, also arranges guided tours for all levels. Phone 360-569-2411 (weekends), 360-569-2271 (midweek).

Olympic National Park, Washington. Guided snowshoe walks are offered at Hurricane Ridge Friday, Saturday, Sunday, and holiday Monday afternoons. Sign up at the Hurricane Ridge Visitor Center for the 1½-hour walk that covers less than a mile. Arboreal highlights include subalpine fir and mountain hemlock. Snowshoe rentals available. Phone 360-565-3131 (recorded park information).

Rocky Mountain National Park, Colorado. Two-hour ranger-guided ecology walks are offered on winter weekends both on the east (Estes Park) and west (Grand Lake) sides of the park and on Wednesdays on the east side. Monthly full-moon walks are also scheduled on the east side. Bring your own snowshoes, or rent them from sporting goods stores in Estes Park or Grand Lake. Phone 970-586-1223 (east side), 970-627-3471 (west side).

Sequoia National Park, California. Guided snowshoe walks and hikes from Wuksachi Village and Lodge are offered on weekends and during holiday midweeks. Rentals available. Phone 559-565-3341.

Yellowstone National Park, Wyoming. A two-hour ranger-led tour along the Riverside Trail into the park leaves from West Yellowstone, Montana. Bring your snowshoes or rent them in town. Phone 406-646-4403. Two-mile, ranger-guided hikes explore the north side of the park. From the Albright Visitor Center at Mammoth Hot Springs, it's a 5- to 15-mile drive to find good snow. Some snowshoes available for complimentary use; rentals also available at a nearby ski shop. Phone 307-344-2263. Additionally, Xanterra Parks & Resorts, the concessionaire that operates Yellowstone hotels and other visitor services, engages naturalist guides who conduct snowshoe tours from the Mammoth Hot Springs Hotel and the Old Faithful Snow Lodge. Snowshoe rentals available. Phone 307-344-7311.

Yosemite National Park, California. The Badger Pass ski area is the winter activities hub, including interpretive snowshoe walks given daily by park rangers. Phone 209-372-0356. Additionally, park concessionaire DNC Parks & Resorts offers guided two-hour moonlight snowshoe walks the night before and the night of each winter full moon. Snowshoes included in the cost. Phone 209-372-1240.

In Canada, abundant snowshoeing opportunities can be found in national, provincial, and city parks and in designated conservation areas, and to an even greater extent than in the United States, Canadian cities and suburbs offer an enormous variety of options for snowshoers. In Quebec City, residents scoot out for a quick snowshoe on the Plains of Abraham in the old walled city as well as on snow-covered paths along the St. Lawrence River. All of the country's 39 national parks lie in the snowbelt, so snowshoeing opportunities abound in the **Parks Canada** jurisdictions. The 14 national parks in the province of Québec are hospitable to snowshoers. For information, go to the Parks Canada Web site (www.parkscanada.gc.ca) or check out www.out-there.com/ssh_m.htm for links to provincial, regional, and local tourism information services. By and large, Canada's national parks are more suited for independent snowshoeing rather than guided excursions, but here are a few interesting options.

Banff National Park, Alberta. "Snowshoe at the Continental Divide" is a daily half-day guided hike through pristine snow-covered forests and along the banks of frozen rivers to track wildlife, learn about winter ecology, and have a snowy good time. Suitable for children eight and older, "Night Tracks" is a 2½-hour program offered four nights a week. The three-hour "Great Divide & Marble Canyon" tour, offered daily, crosses the Continental Divide, as fur traders and natives did in times past. The route follows along Tokumm Creek to Marble Canyon, beneath Mount Whymper, Mount Stanley, and Storm Mountain en route to the snow-blanketed valley beyond. A fourth guided snowshoe hike, called "Explore the Headwaters," leads through a small forest to the source of the Bow River. This three-hour excursion is offered three times a week. Transportation to the trailhead, guide, snowshoes, and poles are included. Phone 877-226-3348 or 403-762-0260. Web site: www.banffinfo.com

Cape Breton Island National Park, Nova Scotia. Sea Scape Outdoor Adventures, located in the whimsically named hamlet of Dingwall, offers daylong guided snowshoe treks into the northern reaches of Cape Breton Highlands National Park, where rugged, rounded hills and wildlife sighting opportunities abound. This outfitter also organizes multi-day packages, including lodging and meals. Phone 902-383-2732. Web site: www.cabot-trail-outdoors.com/winter.html

Jasper National Park, Alberta. Several outfitters based in the town of Jasper conduct guided snowshoe excursions into the park, all including equipment and van transportation to the trailhead. Beyond the Beaten Path offers four-hour guided tours, generally to the Maligne Lake area. Phone 780-852-5650. Walks and Talks Jasper guide Paula Beauchamp's four-hour "Maligne Valley Secrets" tour features a walk on the upper rim of Maligne Canyon. Phone 780-852-4994. The Jasper Adventure Centre takes snowshoers on three-hour tours to Portal Creek, Pyramid Bench, and other areas (depending on snow conditions and wildlife sighting opportunities), and includes equipment and van transport in its tours. Phone 866-952-7737 and 780-852-5595.

SNOWSHOEING ONLINE

You can search for snowshoeing trails scattered across the snowbelt at www.trails.com. This commercial site, which charges an annual fee, is most useful if you want to research other outdoor venues besides snowshoeing sites. Tubbs Snowshoes also maintains a basic trail-finder section on its Web site (tubbssnowshoes.com/trailnet.php). Even better, L. L. Bean, the highly regarded outdoor gear and clothing supplier, maintains an excellent and very international public lands resources Web site. It also has the added benefit of being free of charge. Go to www.llbean.com/parksearch/ and look for snowshoeing sites by location and/or activity.

NORDIC AND ALPINE CENTERS

Marked and maintained trails at most Nordic centers, some Alpine ski areas, and some guest ranches or resort hotels that stay open in winter provide a controlled and comforting environment for snowshoers. While catering to cross-country skiers, many Nordic centers now welcome snowshoers, too. Expect to find day lodges and perhaps trailside warming huts or picnic areas, restrooms, equipment rental, and usually a patrol that comes along at the end of the day to "sweep" the trails and make sure no snowshoers or skiers are still straggling along. Some also offer on-site lodging. These centers generally charge a day-use fee. For information on and links to additional Nordic centers in the United States and Canada, go to the Cross Country Ski Areas Association Web site at www.xcski.org. Alpine ski areas have instituted different snowshoeing policies. Some permit snowshoers on ski trails; others have set aside areas of snowshoeing at the base or on the mountain, sometimes with ski-lift access to the trails. Some charge snowshoers. At others, trail use is free.

SNOWSHOE-FRIENDLY NORDIC CENTERS

THE EAST

The Balsams Wilderness, Dixville Notch, New Hampshire. Landmark luxury lodge known for fine dining, excellent service, and abundant recreational facilities for adults and children. In addition to cross-country trails, the resort has 33 kilometers of snowshoeing trails. Rentals available. Phone 603-255-0600.
Web site: www.thebalsams.com

The Birches Resort, Moosehead Lake, Maine. This snowshoe-friendly, dog-friendly resort on the west shore of Maine's largest lake permits snowshoers on the skating lane of its 40-kilometer Nordic trail system and has an additional 50 kilometers of marked but ungroomed routes that are ideal for snowshoeing. Three yurts for shelter are scattered around the trail system. Guided tours are also available on request. Lodging, meals, and rentals are available, as are such other winter diversions as cross-country skiing, ice fishing, and snowmobiling. Phone 800-823-WILD. Web site: www.birches.com

Bretton Woods, Bretton Woods, New Hampshire. Based on the expansive grounds of the historic and opulent Mount Washington Hotel and the White Mountain National Forest, the 100-kilometer Bretton Woods Nordic network crosses golf courses, spruce and fir glades, beaver ponds and mountain streams, and open hardwood stands. Phone 800-314-1752, 603-278-3320, or 603-278-3322 (Nordic Center). Web site: www.brettonwoods.com

Canterbury Farm Cross Country Ski Center, Becket, Massachusetts. Six trails totaling 10 kilometers lace through a 60-year-old tree farm in the scenic Berkshires, an hour from Albany, New York, two hours from Boston, and four hours from New York City. Rentals available. Phone 412-623-0100. Web site: www.canterbury-farms.com

Five Fields Farm, South Bridgton, Maine. This is a 70-acre working apple orchard that morphs into a dog-friendly cross-country and snowshoeing center between harvest season and apple blossom time. It offers 27 kilometers of trails for snowshoers and skiers, plus virtually unlimited backcountry terrain to the top of scenic Bald Pate Mountain and the surrounding 450-acre land preserve. Phone 207-647-2425. Web site: www.fivefieldsfarmx-cski.com

Hildene Cross-Country Center, Manchester Village, Vermont. This 412-acre historic site is known for the magnificent estate built in 1902 by President Abraham Lincoln's son Robert Todd Lincoln. The carriage barn of the Lincoln family's summer home is transformed into a day lodge during the winter. Snowshoers can share 15 kilometers of trails with cross-country skiers or cavort on three large open fields. Rentals available. Phone 802-362-1788. Web site: www.hildene.org

Jackson Ski Touring Foundation, Jackson, New Hampshire. This organization maintains a huge network of Nordic trails in the shadow of Mount Washington, the mightiest peak in the Northeast. Included in the 69-trail, 155-kilometer system are several snowshoe-specific trails, and snowshoers are also permitted on some, but not all, cross-country trails. The popular guided Snowshoe Instructional Tour, offered almost every Saturday morning, combines an introduction into the natural world with snowshoeing technique tips. Guided snowshoeing is also available by request through the ski school at other times. A demo day is usually held in early to mid-January. Rentals available. Phone 603-383-9355. Web site: www.jacksonxc.org

Lapland Lake Nordic Vacation Center, Northville, New York. Located in the southern region of the 6-million-acre Adirondack Forest Preserve, 60 miles northwest of Albany, the center offers a total of 50 kilometers of scenic, forested trails, 12 kilometers of which are marked and mapped for snowshoeing. Other activities include ice skating, tubing, sledding, and kicksledding, plus a full calendar of special events from November into April. On-site lodging. Rentals available. Phone 518-863-4974 and 800-453-SNOW (snow report). Web site: www.laplandlake.com

Savage River Lodge, Frostburg, Maryland. This small upscale resort in western Maryland, about 2½ hours from Washington, D.C., Baltimore, and Pittsburgh, is the only Nordic center in the state and one of the few in the Mid-Atlantic region. Spread across 800 acres with more than 15 miles of trails, it is suitable for a luxurious weekend getaway or just a day of snowshoeing, with or without a gourmet dinner. The lodge offers guided moonlight snowshoe hikes. Rentals available. Phone 301-689-3200. Web site: www.savageriverlodge.com

Sunday River Inn & Cross Country Ski Center, Newry, Maine. Located just one-half mile from the Sunday River Alpine ski area, the inn has some 50 kilometers of trails, including 12 to 15 kilometers for snowshoeing only — one of which, to the top of Barker Mountain, offers the best views. Guided naturalist tours and fireworks snowshoe tours are available, as well as Tubbs Winter Snowshoe Adventure Day (mid-January) and the riotous April Fools' Pole, Paddle & Paw (late March or early April), a season-transition race of cross-country skiing, canoeing, and snowshoeing with two-person teams competing in costume. Phone 207-824-2410 or 866-232-4354.
Web site: www.sundayriverinn.com

Trapp Family Lodge, Stowe, Vermont. Founded by the famous Austrian expatriate family immortalized in *The Sound of Music,* Trapps' is a pioneering cross-country ski and snowshoeing resort. Snowshoers share 28 ski trails totaling 100 kilometers, including backcountry routes, but also have four trails of their own. The stunning views include Mount Mansfield, the Stowe Valley, and the Worcester Mountain Range. Guided naturalist treks are offered and rentals are available. Phone 800-826-7000 or 802-253-8511.
Web site: www.trappfamily.com

Weston Ski Track, Weston, Massachusetts. This snowmaking-equipped, night-lighted venue is less than 20 (non-rush hour) minutes from Boston with 15 kilometers of trails, including some snowshoeing-only. For new snowshoers, it is a site for Winter Trails Day and also offers the Tubbs Introduction to Snowshoeing package on weekends and holidays. Rentals available. Phone 781-891-6575.
Web site: www.ski-paddle.com

THE MIDWEST

Afterglow Lakes Resort, Phelps, Wisconsin. With some 12 kilometers of marked and packed snowshoeing trails, access to abundant winter trails in the Nicolet National Forest, 11 winterized cabins, and a variety of off-trail activities and amusements, this northern Wisconsin resort is suitable for a few hours or an overnight getaway. Guided snowshoe tours are offered. Rentals available. Phone 715-545-2560. Web site: www.afterglowresort.com

Maplelag Resort, Callaway, Minnesota. This Scandinavian-style resort beside frozen Little Sugarbush Lake is located in a snow pocket about four hours from Minneapolis. Snowshoers are welcome to explore the resort's nearly 660 acres, with more lakes and lovely, gentle scenery. It is the rare resort with convenient commuter air service (to Fargo/Moorhead Airport, one hour away) and proximity to an Amtrak station (Detroit Lakes, less than 20 miles). It offers cabin and lodge accommodations, including a Norwegian log "soddie" moved from a farm near the town of Freeze, Minnesota. Packages include three meals a day and the resort's bottomless cookie jar. Rentals available. Phone 800-654-7711 and 218-375-4466. Web site: www.maplelag.com

Minocqua Winter Park, Minocqua, Wisconsin. Snowshoes may be used on any of Minocqua Winter Park's 74 kilometers of Nordic trails, including the snowshoe-only trails, "Breaking Free" and "Secret Squirrel." Snowshoeing is a big part of the pre-Christmas Silent Sport Demo Days. Rentals available. Phone 715-356-3309.
Web site: www.skimwp.org

Telemark Resort, Cable, Wisconsin. Famous as the start of the American Birkebeiner cross-country ski race, Telemark actually thrives all winter with 200 comfortable condominium units for on-site lodging and direct access to winter trails. The Ojibwa snowshoeing trail is 20 kilometers, segmented into several loops. The resort also holds "candlelight" snowshoe tours and snowshoe races. Phone 715-798-3999 and 877-798-4718. Web site: www.telemarkresort.com

Beaver Meadows Ranch and Resort, Redfeather Lakes, Colorado. In addition to lodging, dining, and an on-property trail system, this resort accesses 25 miles (about 40 kilometers) of adjacent backcountry trails that are ideal for snowshoeing. They are in the woods, sheltered from the wind, and avalanche-free, which is not a trivial matter in northern Colorado. Guided two- or four-hour tours can be arranged for two or more snowshoers. Rentals available. Phone 800-462-5870 or 970-881-2450. Web site: www.beavermeadows.com

Crested Butte Nordic Center, Crested Butte, Colorado. This center, located at Second and Whiterock in downtown Crested Butte, promotes itself as "in town and out of the ordinary." Fourteen shared and exclusive trails totaling 40 kilometers are available. Guided snowshoe walks are available. Special events include the annual Alley Loop Marathon in early February, moonlight snowshoe outings, Progressive Bonfire Dinner in nearby Town Park, and guided backcountry exploration. Rentals available. Phone 970-349-1707. Web site: www.cbnordic.org

Devil's Thumb Ranch, Tabernash, Colorado. This pioneering cross-country center located just north of Winter Park permits snowshoers on most of its 100-kilometer cross-country trail system. There are also 25 to 30 kilometers of snowshoe-only trails. The resort also offers lodging in charming cabins and a top-rated restaurant that serves lunch and dinner. Rentals available. Phone 800-933-4339, 970-726-5632, or 970-726-8231 (Adventure Center).
Web site: www.devilsthumbranch.com

Enchanted Forest Cross Country Ski and Snowshoe Area, Red River, New Mexico. This is the only New Mexico area that offers snowshoe-only trails; it also provides trails shared with skate skiers. It has five trails totaling 15 kilometers and views toward four wilderness areas (including Wheeler Peak, New Mexico's highest mountain). The

monthly Moonlight Snowshoe Tour is a beautiful treat. Rentals available. Phone 505-754-2374 or 800-966-9381.
Web site: www.enchantedforestxc.com

Frisco Nordic Center, Frisco, Colorado. This cross-country center overlooking Lake Dillon boasts 46 kilometers of machine-groomed ski trails with skating lanes snowshoers may use, plus 14 kilometers of snowshoe-only trails laced through the woods. Rentals available. Phone 970-668-0866.
Web site: www.colorado-xc.org/frisco-nordic-center.htm

Galena Lodge/North Valley Trails, Hailey, Idaho. When you think of snowshoeing around storied Sun Valley, the North Valley Trails are where you'll go. Twelve snowshoe-only trails total about 42 kilometers, and snowshoers are required to stay off the cross-country trails. The snowshoe trails, routed through the woods, are designed to showcase views of the Boulder Mountains. Wildlife sightings abound. Local naturalist Cathy Baer guides free, three-hour snowshoe tours. The lodge itself, which dates back to the 1870s, represents a piece of Idaho history. Free shuttle (daily except Monday and Tuesday) from Ketchum/Sun Valley to the Galena Lodge and the trail system. Rentals available. Phone 208-788-2117, 208-726-4010 (Galena Lodge), and 208-726-6662 (trail conditions report).
Web site: www.xcskisv.com/galena.html

Izaak Walton Inn, Essex, Montana. This historic railroad inn at the southern edge of Glacier National Park invites snowshoers to parallel its own 33 kilometers of Nordic trails. It also provides direct access into one of the park's most beguiling winter trails, the Ole Creek trail. The route begins across a short swinging bridge some 15 feet above the frozen creek and winds through forest and along open slopes and rock bluffs. It offers spectacular views of Glacier and into the Great Bear Wilderness west of the inn. Rentals available. Phone 406-888-5700.
Web site: www.izaakwaltoninn.com

Lone Mountain Ranch, Big Sky, Montana. This classic guest ranch adjacent to Montana's preeminent Alpine ski resort boasts an exceptional Nordic center with more than 20 kilometers of dedicated snowshoe trails. Leer Trail boasts awesome views of Lone Peak. Ranch guides lead twice-weekly snowshoe excursions into Yellowstone National Park and also into the Gallatin National Forest backcountry. Lodging, dining, and rentals available. Phone 800-514-4644. Web site: www.lmranch.com

Methow Valley, Winthrop, Washington. This broad valley in north-central Washington boasts three Nordic trail systems connected by the Methow Community Trail, totaling more than 200 kilometers. The "Nature of Winter Series" of interpretive tours (Saturdays throughout the winter, daily on holiday weekends) are led by a local naturalist. The Methow Valley Sport Trails Association, which grooms all the trails, also sponsors a winter-long schedule of special events. Rentals available. Phone 509-996-3287; 800-682-5785 (daily grooming report, Washington only), 509-996-3860 (grooming report), or 509-996-4036 (snowshoe tour information). Web site: www.mvsta.com

Montecito-Sequoia Winter Sports Resort, Los Altos, California. Located off Kings Highway in the Giant Sequoia National Monument between Kings Canyon and Sequoia National Parks, this venue shares the parks' same stunning scenery. Of the 30 kilometers of groomed trails and a total of 90 kilometers of marked trails, snowshoers and skiers share some, while others are dedicated to one or the other activity. Naturalists offer guided snowshoe hikes. Adult and children's rentals available. Phone 800-227-9900 or 559-565-3388. Web site: www.mslodge.com

Snow Mountain Ranch, Granby, Colorado. This vast, informal, and inexpensive family-oriented complex, operated by the YMCA, combines the ambience of a camp with the facilities of a first-rate Nordic and snowshoeing center, with 100 kilometers of trails spread out over

5,100 acres and accommodations for 2,500 in hotel-style rooms and cabins. Rentals available. Guided hikes are offered. Phone 970-887-2152, Ext. 4173 (ski/snowshoe shop). Web site: www.ymcarockies.org

Tamarack Lodge & Resort, Mammoth Lakes, California. This quiet retreat operated by and close to the hot action at Mammoth Mountain is idyllic for snowshoers and ideal for sharing a trip with Alpine skiers or snowboarders. Tamarack features 11 lodge rooms, 31 cabins, a highly regarded lakefront restaurant, and 45 kilometers of groomed trails in the beautiful Lakes Basin, with an adjacent dedicated snowshoeing area. Guided naturalist tours are offered weekly. Rentals available. Phone 800-MAMMOTH or 760-934-2442 (lodge). Web site: www.tamaracklodge.com

White Pine Cross-Country Ski Area, Park City, Utah. White Pine maintains 18 miles of trails overlaid on the local golf course. Touring center staff also lead guided snowshoeing excursions in Empire Canyon at Deer Valley, one of Park City's three downhill ski resorts. The one-hour evening tour, available one night per week, culminates at Deer Valley's classy Empire Canyon Lodge for an opulent fireside dinner. Phone 435-615-5858 (White Pine) or 435-649-1000 (general information). Web sites: www.whitepinetouring.com, www.deervalley.com

CANADA

Hardwood Hills Nordic Ski Centre, Oro Station, Ontario. Located on the rolling Oro Moraine approximately one hour north of Toronto, Hardwood Hills' trails lace through lush forests of deciduous and coniferous trees. "Snowshoeing" should probably be part of its name, too, for it offers 15 kilometers of dedicated snowshoeing trails, plus another kilometer or two shared with cross-country skiers. Rentals available. Phone 705-487-3775 or 800-387-3775 (snow conditions). Web site: www.hardwoodhills.ca

Nipika Mountain Resort, between Radium Hot Springs and Invermere, British Columbia. This backcountry resort at the boundary of Kootenay National Park in the heart of the Canadian Rockies is the place to go for wildlife experiences. A naturalist, who is an expert on wolf biology, conducts animal tracking treks on snowshoes. Elk, deer, wolf, cougar, coyote, and smaller game abound in this area. Additionally, there are 20 kilometers of winter trails. Lodge and cabin accommodations. Phone 877-647-4525 or 250-342-6516. Web site: www.nipika.com

Ski de Fond Mont-Tremblant, Mont Tremblant, Quebec. This Nordic center located between Gray Rocks and Mont Ryan offers 10 kilometers of snowshoe-only trails and puts on a free snowshoe demo day in mid-January, with trail fees and rental charges waived. The center has three warming areas and a snack bar serving healthful food. Rentals available. Phone 819-425-5588.
Web site: www.skidefondmont-tremblant.com

Stokely Creek Lodge, Goulais River, Ontario. Located 20 miles north of Sault Ste. Marie, this classic lodge and touring center boasts 130 kilometers of stunning trails. Most of the trails are at a modest elevation, but one ascends King Mountain, which at 1,880 feet is the region's highest peak. Views extend to the Algoma Highlands and Haviland Bay on Lake Superior's eastern shore. Rentals available. Phone 866-786-5359 or 705-649-3421.
Web site: www.stokelycreek.com

Wye Marsh Wildlife Centre, Midland, Ontario. The Wye Valley north of Toronto is a wildlife management area inhabited by deer, coyotes, fox, beaver, and many more mammals, as well as winter birds and trumpeter swans. Along the 22 kilometers of winter trails interpretive signage explains the valley's landforms and wildlife. Weekly interpretive snowshoe walks are offered. Rentals available. Phone 705-526-7809. Web site: www.wyemarsh.com

SNOWSHOEING AT ALPINE SKI RESORTS

Bolton Valley, Vermont. In addition to a Nordic center with a one and three-quarter-mile designated snowshoe and dog trail, this compact, family-oriented resort in northern Vermont sits at the doorstep to about 5,200 forested acres, the largest area of protected and preserved back-country land of any New England ski resort, with numerous trails and loops and two backcountry cabins available for both day and overnight use. Bolton offers four guided snowshoe excursions, including a beginner tour and a kids' tour. Rentals available. Phone 802-434-3444. Web site: www.boltonvalley.com

Loon Mountain, New Hampshire. This Alpine resort in the Mount Washington area has an adjacent 37-kilometer network of snowshoer-friendly cross-country trails. Rental equipment is available at the Adventure Center, located across from the main parking lot. Phone 603-745-6281, Ext. 5562 (Adventure Center). Web site: www.loonmtn.com

Okemo, Ludlow, Vermont. This exceptionally welcoming resort permits snowshoers on 5 kilometers of trails on the periphery of Okemo Mountain and also on 10 kilometers of dedicated snowshoe trails at the Okemo Valley Nordic Center. On selected holiday evenings, guided snowshoe treks head up the mountain for unbeatable views of the fireworks. Rentals available. Phone 802-228-4041 (general information) or 802-228-1396 (Nordic center). Web site: www.okemo.com

Smugglers' Notch, Vermont. Twenty kilometers of dedicated snowshoe trails wander through the woods beyond Morse Mountain, one of three interlinked Alpine ski mountains. The popular Adventure Dinner includes an early-evening lift ride to the Sterling Mountain summit, a guided snowshoe outing, and a candlelight dinner. Snowshoeing is part of the resort's annual Heritage WinterFest in late January. Smugglers' Notch also hosts the Northern Vermont Snowshoe Challenge in mid-February, comprising a 5-kilometer run and a 2-kilometer walk. Phone 800-451-8752 or 802-644-8851. Web site: www.smuggs.com

Stratton Mountain, Vermont. There are two Nordic Centers, one at the Country Club and one on the mountain at the Sun Bowl. Snowshoers are not restricted from any of the 30 kilometers of Nordic trails. Additional attractions are a summit snowshoe trek to an old fire tower, guided nature tours, a moonlight hike to the Pearl S. Buck Stone House, and the annual Owl Prowl, an evening snowshoe excursion to the Vermont Raptor Center. Phone 802-297-4114.
Web site: www.stratton.com

Sugarbush, Vermont. In addition to marked snowshoe trails at Lincoln Peak, the resort offers guided evening snowshoe tours of easy trails and also twice-daily of steeper, more rigorous Slide Brook Basin on selected weekend and holiday dates. Rentals are available (and included in tours), weather and conditions permitting. A nearby outfitter called Vermont Pack & Paddle also offers full-moon tours to a remote cabin for an opulent dinner feast. Rentals available. Phone 800-53-SUGAR (reservations and general information) or 802-583-6537 (guest services for snowshoeing tours). Web site: www.sugarbush.com

Sugarloaf/USA, Maine. Snowshoeing is permitted on the skating lanes of the entire, vast 100-kilometer trail system that includes 11 kilometers of snowshoeing-only trails and access to a trailside solar-heated warming hut. The trails weave through the beautiful, forested Longfellow Mountains. Shoe & Stew is a women-only, midweek tour followed by a hearty, sit-down stew lunch at the Klister Kitchen. Moonlight snowshoe hikes are also offered. Phone 800-THE-LOAF (reservations), 207-237-2000 (general information), or 207-237-6808 (snow phone). Web site: www.sugarloaf.com

THE MIDWEST

Boyne Mountain and Boyne Highlands, Michigan. Between 25 and 35 kilometers of Nordic trails at each resort are groomed and packed wide for classical cross-country skiing, skating, and snowshoeing. Snowshoers may go anywhere except on the classical tracks. The terrain ranges from flat to hilly, with interesting climbs and descents. Trail maps and rentals are available. Phone 231-549-6088 (Boyne Nordican) or 231-526-3029 (Boyne Highlands Cross-Country Center).

Giants Ridge, Biwabik, Minnesota. In addition to Alpine skiing and Nordic trails, this ski resort boasts the exceptional Sleeping Giant snowshoe trail, which is four miles long and climbs to the top of the Laurentian Divide, affording wonderful views. Rentals available. Phone 800-688-7669. Web site: www.giantsridge.com

THE WEST

Angel Fire, New Mexico. The resort's scenic Nordic trails are on top of the mountain. Snowshoers carry their equipment and board the Chile Express Chairlift to trail access at 10,650 feet. The four marked trails total 22 kilometers, ranging from an easy 2.6-kilometer loop to a challenging 9.8 kilometers. At the end of the hike, snowshoers download on the chairlift. Rentals available. Phone 888-472-0124 (reservations) or 505-377-4273 (general information).
Web site: www.angelfireresort.com

Aspen Mountain, Colorado. The lifts and downhill trails are actually the north-facing prow of a long ridge. The Aspen Center for Environmental Studies conducts one of its three snowshoeing tours from the summit southward along Richmond Ridge. It is also possible to buy a single foot-passenger gondola ticket and snowshoe independently. Aspen Mountain phone 800-308-6936 or 970-925-1220.
Web site: www.aspensnowmass.com. ACES phone 970-925-7345.
Web site: www.aspennature.org

Beaver Creek, Avon, Colorado. An ultra-classy Alpine resort that has a 32-kilometer trail system comprising both groomed and rustic routes, a warming hut, and several trailside picnic spots and yurts. You can snowshoe a groomed and signed 8-kilometer trail between the lodging centers of Beaver Creek Village, Bachelor Gulch Village, and Arrowhead Village. Beaver Creek also offers guided naturalist excursions and hosts snowshoe races and special events during the season. Rentals available. Phone 970-845-5313. Web site: www.beavercreek.com

Crested Butte, Colorado. In addition to snowshoeing options available at the in-town Crested Butte Nordic Center (see page 111), the Alpine ski area welcomes snowshoers with two on-mountain tours. Guided morning and afternoon snowshoe walks offered daily include a ride up the Keystone lift to trails that are surprisingly secluded and offer beautiful views toward Gothic. Monthly moonlight tours include a snowcat ride up the mountain, followed by a guided snowshoe walk back down to the base area for hot chocolate or ice cream. Rentals available (and included in the cost of the moonlight tour). Phone 888-223-2631 (ask for Guest Services). Web site: www.skicb.com

Grand Targhee, Wyoming. Snowshoeing is permitted on the 15-kilometer Nordic network that winds through the woods and over the meadows at the base of this small resort that nestles on the west side of the monumental peak called the Grand Teton. The resort's naturalist conducts twice-daily, two-hour interpretive tours Thursday through Sunday. Phone 800-TARGHEE. Web site: www.grandtarghee.com

Kirkwood, California. At this winter resort south of Lake Tahoe, Nordic skiing is the peer of Alpine, and snowshoers are welcome on all of the 80 kilometers of marked cross-country trails. Two of the trails are dog-friendly as well as snowshoer-friendly. Among them, Kirkwood's three interconnected trail systems feature two trailheads, three warming huts, and great views. "Soup and Shoe" is a monthly guided snowshoe excursion to the crest of the ridge above Kirkwood, rewarded by hot hearty soup and bread. "Night Walking" is a monthly full-moon tour. Phone 209-258-7248. Web site: www.kirkwood.com

Northstar-at-Tahoe, Twin Bridges, California. This family-oriented resort has established its Nordic Ski and Snowshoe Center at mid-mountain, with access to 50 kilometers of groomed trails separate from the downhill runs. Full-moon snowshoe tours are a monthly treat. Rentals available. Phone 800-Go-NORTH.
Web site: www.NorthstarAtTahoe.com

Steamboat, Colorado. This huge northern Colorado mountain permits limited snowshoeing on some of its downhill runs. Three snowshoeing trails of various lengths and pitches are all accessible from Thunderhead atop the gondola, also the jumping-off point for half-day, full-day, and moonlight guided snowshoeing tours, including the gourmet lunch tour that culminates at Ragnar's Restaurant. Additionally, the nearby Steamboat Touring Center has a 5-kilometer dedicated snowshoe trail. Phone 970-879-0740, 970-871-5191, or 800-922-2722.
Web site: www.steamboat.com

Telluride, Colorado. Join a scenic, guided snowshoe tour from the Topaten Touring Center, at the top of Lift 10. The views of Prospect Bowl, Magic Meadows, and the soaring San Juan Mountains all around make it a memorable excursion. Phone 970-728-7517.
Web site: www.tellurideskiresort.com

Winter Park, Colorado. Easy, two-hour on-mountain snowshoe tours are offered twice daily and include a short chairlift ride followed by a gentle downhill tramp through dense woods to the base. For those seeking a more vigorous workout, the resort's Advanced Adventure Snowshoe Tours, offered Saturdays and Sundays, are 3½ hours and five miles of challenging up-and-down terrain. Tours include rentals. Phone 970-726-5514, 303-892-0961 (Denver), or 970-726-SNOW (snow conditions). Web site: www.skiwinterpark.com

Cypress Mountain, British Columbia. In addition to 10 kilometers of dedicated snowshoeing routes from a separate Nordic base near the Alpine ski area, Cypress offers two-hour guided naturalist tours several times a week, guided three-hour evening tours for women only, and a sensational fondue tour six nights a week, culminating in a fine dinner in the rustic ambience of historic lakeside Hollyburn Lodge. Cypress's walk/run clinics for snowshoers who want to increase their fitness level are popular with athletes from nearby Vancouver. Phone 604-922-0825 (Nordic center). Web site: www.cypressmountain.com

Mont Sainte-Anne, Quebec. Five marked trails bordering this sprawling Alpine ski area near Quebec City total 30 kilometers and are accessed free of charge for independent snowshoeing. Additionally, the ski area offers a brief mountaintop snowshoe walk from the top of the gondola to the cozy and charming La Crête Lodge for a fondue dinner. Phone 800-463-1568 or 418-827-5281.
Web site: www.mont-sainte-anne.com

Mount Washington Alpine Resort, Vancouver Island, British Columbia. This thriving resort offers on-site accommodations for 3,500 guests in log cabins and condominiums. Of the 55 kilometers of groomed trails woven through the 2,000-acre property and in adjacent Strathcona Provincial Park, 20 kilometers are for snowshoeing only. The Friday night Snowshoe Fondue is an evening guided snowshoe followed by a fondue supper. The resort also hosts the Atlas Snowshoe Romp, a family event, and "The Yeti," Canada's first snowshoe race series. Rentals available. Phone 250-338-1386 or 888-231-1499.
Web site: www.mountwashington.ca

Silver Star, British Columbia. This delightful Alpine resort, with excellent family programs and a 55-kilometer cross-country trail system, also offers organized snowshoeing. Programs include the Sunset Snowshoe Adventure, a guided two-hour walk along a historic trail with spectacular views to watch the sunset, and Chocolate Dreams, a three-hour evening excursion that offers chocolate fondue and a sleigh ride. Beverages and/or snacks, plus headlamps for the three after-dark hikes, and snowshoe rentals are included. Phone 800-663-4431 or 250-542-0224. Web site: www.skisilverstar.com

Sun Peaks, British Columbia. Along this resort's 12 kilometers of designated snowshoe trails are bird-feeding stations, wildlife-viewing areas, and even a snow cave. Birds that overwinter in this area include ruffed grouse, red-tail hawks, black-capped chickadees, blue and gray jays, bald eagles and peregrine falcons. Two-hour guided interpretive tours, offered in the afternoon and evening, include nature and history at and around the resort, plus hot apple cider and a snack. Rentals available. Phone 800-807-3257 or 250-578-5542.
Web site: www.sunpeaksresort.com

Whistler, British Columbia. Canada's largest year-round resort and best-known ski destination also offers unsurpassed snowshoeing opportunities. On-mountain tours begin daily and accommodate various levels of snowshoers. Nature and dinner tours are offered. Phone 604-904-7060. Web site: www.whistelerblackcomb.com. It is possible to hike along valley trails or join one of several guided tours that can be booked through the Whistler Activity and Outdoor Information Centre, located in the Whistler Conference Centre. Phone 877-991-9988 or 604-938-2769. Web site: www.mywhistler.com. Among the guide services offering snowshoeing tours, Blackcomb Snowshoe stands out for its evening tour to Mallard Mountain and its fondue dinner excursion. Phone 604-932-6681. Callaghan Country Wilderness Adventures transports guests for a full-day excursion to a remote backcountry lodge, where snowshoers can explore old-growth forests and subalpine meadows. Phone 604-938-0656.
Web site: www.callaghancountry.com

A RACE SAMPLER

Nationwide, there seem to be more and more races, bigger ones and better ones every year. Most races require an entry fee and offer an array of awards and prizes at the end. Beyond those basics, there is great variety in the style and seriousness of the races. Pre-registration is usually recommended, though most races also offer same-day registration. Most races have men's and women's divisions, and many are also divided into age categories. Many events include a family or fun category so that children can also participate. Here is a sampling of snowshoe races across the continent.

SEASON-LONG SERIES

Beaver Creek Snowshoe Adventure Series. Beaver Creek, Colorado. One of the nation's premier snowshoeing series, with monthly competitions. Top racers go to the North American Snowshoe Championships. 10K run, 5K run/walk, and kids' 1K race. Phone 970-476-6797. Web site: www.gohighline.com/bcsnowshoe/

Empire State Snowshoe Racing Association (ESSRA) Series. Roughly three dozen snowshoe races in New York State, mostly sprint and 5K distances. Some are qualifiers for the Winter Empire State Games. Phone 518-643-8806 (evenings).
Web site: www.dionsnowshoes.com/essnowshoera.html

Maine Snowshoe Series. Four races in January and February, from 2 to 10K. Web site: www.dionsnowshoes.com/masnse.html

Mount Hood Snowshoe Series, Oregon. Three events: White River 8K, a classic competition that also has a 2K recreational component;

Frog Lake 5-mile; and Iron Creek Winter Duathlon, comprising a 5K snowshoe race followed by an optional 5K cross-country ski leg. Phone 503-497-4080.
Web site: www.xdogevents.com/html/snowshoe_series.html

Salomon Nordic Series. Four cross-country ski competitions, each in a different Colorado location, each with a 5K snowshoe race. Phone 303-635-2815. Web site: www.emgcolorado.com

United States National Snowshoe Champion Series. Elite series with nine regional qualifiers throughout the season in each of five United States regions (Alaskan, Western, Rocky Mountain, North Central, and Northeast) at 5K and 10K distances. Finale is the United States National Snowshoe Championships held each March at different locations. Some qualifiers themselves are series, such as the Bigfoot Snowshoe Race held at several Midwestern venues on the same day in January and other regional series in this section. Phone 518-643-8806. Web site: www.snowshoeracing.com

Western Massachusetts Athletic Club Snowshoe Race Series. Fourteen race days weekly from December through mid-March in western Massachusetts, Vermont, and New York State. Distances range from 5K to 15K, and sometimes two distances are scheduled for the same day and location. Web site: www.runwmac.com

Yeti Mountain Snowshoe Series. 5K and 10K races for beginning and advanced competitors at resorts across British Columbia. Phone 604-738-0217. Web site: www.theyeti.ca

DECEMBER

Day of Infamy Snowshoe Race. Glenwood Springs, Colorado. Annual Pearl Harbor Day 8K race in Babbish Gulch. Phone 970-876-0683 or 970-379-2593. Web site: www.dayofinfamysnowshoerace.org.

Off-Track, Off-Beat Snowshoe Race. Leadville, Colorado. High-altitude racing season opener. 10K on unset, ungroomed, untracked routes that require navigation skills as well as endurance.
Phone 719-539-4112. Web site: www.racingunderground.com

Rail Trail Snowshoe Stomp. Park City, Utah. 5K race that takes place along rails-to-trails Union Pacific right of way.
Phone 801-583-6281.
Web site: www.sports-am.com

Red Butte Snowshoe Run. Salt Lake City, Utah. 5K and family fun event at Red Butte Gardens. Phone 801-583-6281.
Web site: www.sports-am.com

Turquoise Lake 20K Snowshoe Run. Leadville, Colorado. Endurance race with 2,700 feet of elevation gain. Phone 719-539-4112. Web site: www.racingunderground.com

JANUARY

MVSTA Mazama Snowshoe Demo. Winthrop, Washington. Demo day includes 2K, 5K, and 10K races. Phone 509-996-3287.
Web site: www.mvsta.com

Perkinstown Tramp. Perkinstown, Wisconsin. 5K, 10K, Mountaineer, and kids' fun categories. Mountaineer competitors must use large snowshoes (10 by 46 inches for men on the 10K course and 8 by 25 inches for women on the 5K course) and carry a 15-pound pack.
Phone 715-267-6266. Web site: www.perkinstowntramp.com

Romp to Stomp Out Breast Cancer. Stratton, Vermont. Also known as the Komen Vermont–New Hampshire Race for the Cure.
Web site: www.stratton.com

FEBRUARY

Alley Loop. Crested Butte, Colorado. 10K snowshoe race (and cross-country ski races at various distances) through the alleys of this historic town. Phone 970-349-1707. Web site: www.cbnordic.org

Badger State Games. Competitions in various Wisconsin locations. 4 by 100 and 4 by 200 relays, 1-mile and 5K runs, children's fun run, mountaineer, and 5-mile run/tour. Phone 608-226-4780.
Web site: www.sportswisconsin.com

Book Across The Bay. Ashland to Washburn, Wisconsin. 10K race across Lake Superior's Chequamegon Bay. The route is lighted by *luminarias.* Phone 800-284-9484. Web site: www.batb.org

Frozen Toe Tromp and Glide. Tabernash, Colorado. Women's 5K snowshoe race, recreational race, and cross-country ski racing at Devil's Thumb Ranch Resort. Phone 970-725-3442.
Web site: www.gcadvocates.org

Gold Rush. Frisco, Colorado. 5K snowshoe race (and cross-country ski at various distances) at Frisco Nordic Center. Phone 303-635-2815.

Grouse Mountain Snowshoe Classic (formerly called Dam Bigfoot Snowshoe Challenge). Grouse Mountain, British Columbia. 5K and 10K races; 2.5K kids' event. Phone 604-980-9311.
Web site: www.grousemountain.com

Jordanelle Snowshoe Race. Jordanelle State Park, Utah. 5K race and family fun events. Phone 801-583-6281.
Web site: www.sports-am.com

Mosquito Hill Snowshoe Races. New London, Wisconsin. 1-, 3-, and 6-mile races for all ages; 200 meter kids' race. Phone 920-779-6433.

Mother of All Ascensions. Snowmass, Colorado. Uphill race at the Snowmass ski area. Phone 970-923-2000, Ext. 210. Web site: www.snowmassvillage.com

Mount Taylor Winter Quadrathlon. Grants, New Mexico. Bike 13 miles, run 5 miles, ski 3 miles, and snowshoe 1 mile to the top of 11,400-foot Mount Taylor, then reverse the order back down to the town of Grants for a total distance of 44 miles. Phone 800-748-2142 or 505-287-4802. Web site: http://mttaylorquad.org

New World Snowshoe Championship. Luck, Wisconsin. 5K, 10K, and 20K races. Phone 715-472-8231.

Screamin' Snowman Snowshoe Race. Eldora Resort Nordic Center, Colorado. 5K and 10K runs, 1-mile fun walk. Phone 303-642-7917. Web site: www.racingunderground.com/sssnowman.html

Swift Skedaddle. Frisco, Colorado. 3K and 10K races at the Frisco Nordic Center. Phone 970-389-4838.

Wild Hare Snowshoe Race and Trek. Tabernash, Colorado. 5K women's race at Devil's Thumb Ranch Resort. Phone 303-316-8392. Web site: www.thesportingwoman.com

Yukon Arctic Ultra. Whitehorse, Yukon Territory. Extremely demanding endurance race under severe winter conditions with 100K and 300K options. Competitors start on the Yukon Quest route after the dogsled teams take off. They may run, ski, or bike; those in the "running" category have the option of using snowshoes. Phone 44+ 1753-687517. Web sites: www.eventrate.com and www.4ar.info/rdt/yukonarcticultra/index.php

MARCH

America's Uphill. Aspen, Colorado. Begins at the base of Little Nell, ascends 3,267 feet up Aspen Mountain, and finishes at 11,212 feet. Phone 970-925-2849. Web site: www.utemountaineer.com

Big Sky Winterfest. Big Sky, Montana. Fun-filled day including various cross-country ski and snowshoe races. Phone 406-995-5000. Web site: www.bigskyresort.com

Hula Moon Snowshoe Classic. Durango Mountain Resort, Colorado. 5K snowshoe race. Starts under a full moon and follows a loop course lined by tiki torches and glow sticks. Phone 970-385-8901, Ext. 111. Web site: www.durangomountainresort.com

Steamboat Pentathlon. Steamboat Springs, Colorado. Multi-sport event with long and short courses. Ski or snowboard down 400 vertical feet of Howelsen Hill, snowshoe 1½ or 3 miles, cross-country ski 4½ or 2¼ miles, mountain bike 12 or 7.4 miles, and run 5 or 2 miles. Phone 970-879-4300. Web site: www.ci.steamboat.co.us

Susan G. Komen Tubbs Snowshoe Fundraiser. Frisco, Colorado. 5K run and 3K walk at the Frisco Nordic Center. Phone 970-668-0866.

APRIL

Hidden Peak Snowshoe Hill Climb. Snowbird, Utah. Spring ascent up the slopes of the Snowbird ski resort with 3,000 feet of elevation gain. Phone 801-583-6281. Web site: www.sports-am.com

Snowshoe Shuffle. Vail, Colorado. The largest snowshoe event in the United States. Competitive 10K race, competitive and recreational 5K races, and 1-mile snowshoe "stroll." Phone 970-569-7485. Web site: www.snowshoeshuffle.com

SNOWSHOE SOURCES

Snowshoe manufacturers and distributors have been coming (with the upwelling of the sport's popularity) and going (with the stiff competition and increasing market saturation). But here are the snowshoeing companies currently distributing their products in North America.

Arctic Trekker Snowshoe
(See Industrial Reproductions Ltd.)

Atlas Snow-Shoe Company*
115 Tenth Street
San Francisco, CA 94103
Phone: 888-48-ATLAS
  or 415-703-0414
Web site:
  www.atlassnowshoe.com

Baldas Snowshoes
1101 Wetherburn
Winston-Salem, NC 27104
Web site: www.baldas.com

**C3-Design Innovations
(Verts snowshoes)**
6146 South 350 West
Salt Lake City, UT 84107
Phone: 801-281-1331
Web site: www.verts.com

**Cascade Toboggan
Company
(Powder-Wings snowshoes)**
1808 Industrial Drive
Sandpoint, ID 83864
Phone: 208-263-2484
  or 800-453-1192
Web site:
www.cascadetoboggan.com
*Snowshoes, backcountry
camping, rescue and first-aid
products*

Crescent Moon Snowshoes
1190 Crestmoor
Boulder, CO 80303
Phone: 303-494-5506
  or 800-587-7655
Web site:
www.crescentmoonsnow-shoes.com
*Snowshoes, poles, traction
systems, snowshoe bags,
booties, gaiters*

Denali snowshoes
(See Mountain Safety
Research)

Dion Snowshoes
397 Ross Road
Readsboro, VT 05350
Phone: 802-423-7537
Web site:
  www.dionsnowshoes.com
*Snowshoes, build-your-own
snowshoe kits*

**Due North
(GV Snowshoes)**
11345 Highway 17 West
Sturgeon Falls, Ontario
P2B 3K7, Canada
Phone: 877-258-4180 or
  705-753-2387
*Snowshoes (wood-frame and
contemporary materials)*

**Faber and Company
Snowshoes**
180 Rue de la Rivière
Loretteville, Québec
G2B 3W6, Canada
Phone: 418-842-8476
Web site:
www.fabersnowshoes.com

Glacier Snowshoes
5910 Durrerin Drive
Savage, MN 55378
Phone: 952-440-6262
Web site:
www.glaciersnowshoe.com

Grivel Mont Blanc
11013 Courmayeur Mont
Blanc, Aosta
Italy
Phone: +39.0165.84.37.14
Fax: +39.0165.84.48.00
E-mail: info@grivel.com
Web site: www.grivel.com
*Snowshoes, mountaineering
and ice climbing equipment*

GV Snowshoes
(See Due North)

Havlick Snowshoes
2513 State Highway 30,
Drawer QQ
Mayfield, NY 12117
Phone: 800-867-7463
  or 518-661-4644
Web site:
www.havlicksnowshoe.com
*Snowshoes, poles, bindings
for traditional snowshoes*

Industrial Reproductions Ltd. (Arctic Trekker snowshoes)
610 Richard Road
Prince George, British
Columbia V2K-4L3
Canada
Phone: 800-663-6843
Web site: www.irl.bc.ca

InSTEP Snowshoes
4902 Hammersley Road
Madison, WI 53711
Phone: 800-242-6110
Web site: www.instep.net
Snowshoes, collapsible snow shovels, children's plastic snowshoes

Iverson Snowshoe Company
85 Maple Street,
P.O. Box 85
Shingleton, MI 49884
Phone: 906-452-6370
Web site: www.iversonsnowshoe.com
Wood-frame snowshoes

LEKI USA
356 Sonwil Drive
Buffalo, NY 14225
Phone: 800-255-9982
Web site: www.leki.com
Poles

Life-Link International
P.O. Box 2913
1240 Huff Lane
Jackson, WY 83001
Phone: 800-443-8620
Web site:
www.life-link.com
Poles, shovels, snow-safety, emergency, and avalanche equipment

Little Bear Snowshoes* (children's snowshoes)
1110 Kimball Avenue
Grand Junction, CO 81501
Phone: 800-655-8984 or
970-241-8546
Web site: www.little-bearsnowshoes.com

Lowa Boots
86 Viaduct Road
Stamford, CT 06907
Phone: 203-353-0116
Web site:
www.lowaboots.com
Snowshoes, boots

Merrell Footwear
9341 Courtland Drive NE
Rockford, MI 49351
Phone: 800-789-8586
Web site:
www.merrellboot.com
Waterproof insulated boots

Michigan Snowshoe Center
522 North Fifth Street
Roscommon, MI 48653
Phone: 866-275-0300
or 989-275-0300
Web site: www.snowshoecenter.com
Build-your-own snowshoe kits

Montana Snowshoes (Yeti snowshoes)
1409 South 600 West,
Suite D
Bountiful, UT 84010
Phone: 801-298-0476
Web site: www.snowstuf.com
Snowshoes, emergency and survival products, backpacks

Mountain Safety Research (Denali snowshoes)
4000 First Avenue South,
P.O. Box 24547
Seattle, WA 98134
Phone: 800-531-9531
or 206-505-9500
Web site: www.msrgear.com
Snowshoes, poles, heavy-duty camping equipment

Northern Lites Snowshoes
300 South 86th Avenue
Wausau, WI 54401
Phone: 800-360-LITE
Web site:
www.northernlites.com

PowderWings
(See Cascade Toboggan Company)

Prater Snowshoes
3740 Cove Road
Ellensburg, WA 98926
Phone: 509-925-1212
Web site:
www.adsnet.net/prater

Redfeather Snowshoes
4705-A Oakland Street
Denver, CO 80239
Phone: 800-525-0081
or 303-375-0410
Web site:
www.redfeather.com

Sherpa Snowshoe Company
9640 South 60th Street
Franklin, WI 53132
Phone: 800-621-2277
Web site:
www.sherpasnowshoes.com

TSL Sport Equipment
(See Lowa Boots, former distributor in the United States)
Web site: www.tslsportequipment.com
Snowshoes, bindings, poles, footwear, headlamps

Tubbs Snowshoes*
52 River Road,
P.O. Box 1319
Stowe, VT 05672
Phone: 800-882-2748
  or 802-253-7398
Web site:
  www.tubbssnowshoes.com

Ursus Snowshoes
2019 East Seventh Avenue
Vancouver, British Columbia
V5N 1S5, Canada
Phone: 604-254-4517

Verts snowshoes
(See C3-Design Innovations)

Wilcox & Williams (Country Ways)
6001 Lyndale Avenue South
Minneapolis, MN 55419
Phone: 800-216-0710
  or 612-861-2262
Web site:
  www.snowshoe.com
Wood-frame snowshoes, make-your-own snowshoe kits, snowshoe furniture, how-to videos

Yakima Snowshoes
1385 8th Street
Arcata, CA 95521
Phone: 888-925-0703 or
  707-826-8000
Web site: www.yakima.com

Yeti Snowshoes
(See Montana Snowshoes)

Yowie Snowshoes Pty. Ltd.
122 Kororoit Creek Road
Williamstown, Victoria
3016, Australia
Phone: +61 3 9397 2115
E-mail: info@yowies.com.au
Web site:
  www.yowies.com.au

Yukon Charlie's Winter Systems
52 Gunning Point Road
Plymouth, MA 02360
Phone: 866-SNO-SHOE
Web site:
  www.yukoncharlies.com
Snowshoes, poles, snowshoe gear bags

* These three companies have recently come under new ownership. It is likely that some locations will close or consolidate, but at this writing, all three brands are supposed to continue. Toll-free phone numbers and Web sites will most likely also remain in place.

ONLINE SNOWSHOE SOURCES

Below are online retailers with a brick-and-mortar presence and a long track record of customer service, as well as well-established catalog/online merchants.

L. L. Bean
www.llbean.com

Cabela's
www.cabelas.com

Campmor
www.campmor.com

Early Winters
www.earlywinters.com

Eastern Mountain Sports (EMS)
www.ems.com

Piragis Northwest Company (a.k.a., Boundary Waters Catalog)
www.piragis.com

Recreation Equipment Inc. (REI)
www.rei.com

Title 9 Sports (women's equipment and clothing)
www.title9sports.com

Sierra Trading Post
www.sierratradingpost.com

ORGANIZATIONS

The following outdoor-recreation organizations organize group snowshoe hikes and treks. Some also operate winterized backcountry cabins accessible on snowshoes.

Adirondack Mountain Club
814 Goggins Road
Lake George, NY 12845
Phone: 518-668-4447
or 800-395-8080
Web site: www.adk.org

Alpine Club of Canada
P. O. Box 8040
Indian Flats Road
Canmore, Alberta T1W 2T8, Canada
Phone: 403-678-3200
Web site:
www.alpineclubofcanada.ca

American Hiking Society
1422 Fenwick Lane
Silver Spring, MD 20910
Phone: 301-565-6704
Web site:
www.americanhiking.org

Appalachian Mountain Club
5 Joy Street
Boston, MA 02108
Phone: 617-523-0636
Web site: www.outdoors.org

Backcountry Snowsports Alliance
P.O. Box 3067
Eldorado Springs, CO 80025
Phone: 303-494-5266
Web site: http://backcountryalliance.org

Colorado Mountain Club
710 10th Street
Golden, CO 80401
Phone: 303-279-3080
Web site: www.cmc.org

Green Mountain Club
4711 Waterbury-Stowe Rd.
Waterbury Center, VT 05677
Phone: 802-244-7037
Web site: www.greenmountainclub.org

Mazamas
909 NW 19th Avenue
Portland, OR 97209
Phone: 503-227-2345
Web site:
www.mazamas.org

The Mountaineers
300 Third Avenue West
Seattle, WA 98119
Phone: 206-284-6310
Web site:
www.mountaineers.org

Sierra Club
85 Second Street, 2nd Floor
San Francisco, CA 94105
Phone: 415-977-5500
Web site:
www.sierraclub.org

United States Snowshoe Association
678 County Route 25
Corinth, New York 12822
Phone: 518-654-7648
Web site:
www.snowshoeracing.com

OTHER ONLINE RESOURCES

www.nps.gov
The National Park Service site offers links to individual park sites with lists of activities.

www.fs.fed.us
The United States Forest Service offers the most extensive network of marked winter trails in the country.

www.parkscanada.ca
Parks Canada is the agency that protects and manages the country's vast national parks system.

www.audubon.org
The National Audubon Society offers interpretive snowshoeing tours.

www.wintertrails.org
The Winter Trails Day site offers schedules and more.

www.awg.org
Information about the Arctic Winter Games.

http://maps.nationalgeographic.com/trails/
National Geographic offers the National Geographic Trails Illustrated series of maps.

www.gemtrek.com
Maps for the Canadian Rockies.

www.snowshoemag.com
An on-line magazine for snowshoeing enthusiasts.

INDEX

Pages with illustrations are *italicized.*

OTHER STOREY TITLES YOU WILL ENJOY

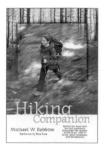

The Hiking Companion, by Michael W. Robbins. Including discussions of common mistakes and how to avoid them, recommendations on trip planning and equipment, and lessons on basic navigation, as well as exciting stories of once-in-a-lifetime adventures, *The Hiking Companion* is a perfect reader for the millions of hiking enthusiasts. 136 pages. Paperback. ISBN 1-58017-429-9

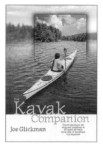

The Kayak Companion, by Joe Glickman. Joe Glickman, a two-time member of the U.S. National Marathon Kayak Team, teaches beginners the basic techniques of sea, touring, and recreational kayaking, and offers expert advice on navigation, troubleshooting, and boat assessment to more experienced kayakers. Woven throughout the narrative are Glickman's stories of his own kayaking adventures. 136 pages. Paperback. ISBN 1-58017-485-X